The Outback Diaries

By

Randy Tharp

The Outback Diaries

Randy Tharp

Published by Randy Tharp, 2024.

While every precaution has been taken in the preparation of this book, the publisher assumes no responsibility for errors or omissions, or for damages resulting from the use of the information contained herein.

THE OUTBACK DIARIES

First edition. March 20, 2024.

Copyright © 2024 Randy Tharp.

ISBN: 979-8224000241

Written by Randy Tharp.

Table of Contents

Dedication

Dementia, senility, and all other ailments associated with cognitive decline are lousy awful bad.

This one goes out to all of those who have experienced loss of the mind, whether it's directly, eventually, or in the orbit of a loved one.

On a more personal note, I dedicate this to the woman who gave me this story in the first place.

This is for my mother Barb.

We miss you and love you very much.

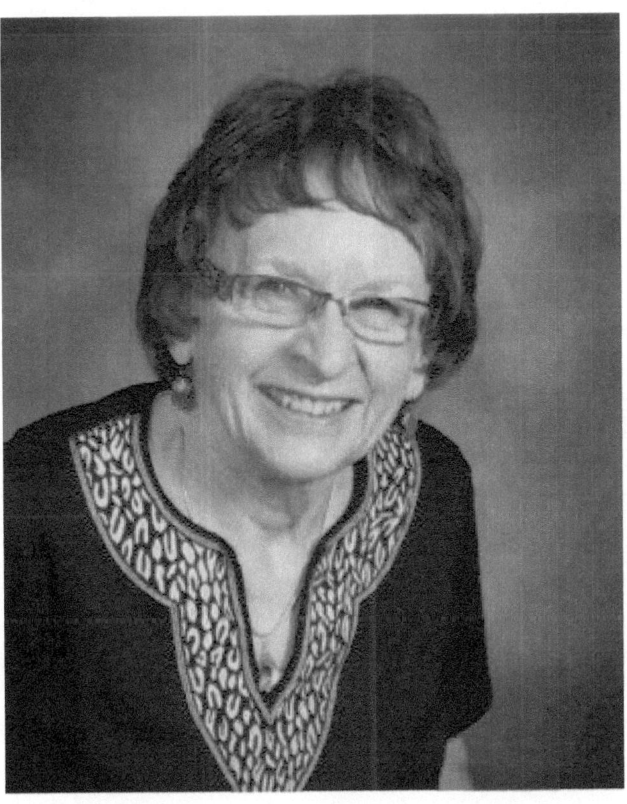

Forward

There's something to be said for writing a letter to yourself and addressing it to some point in the past.

It's difficult.

The formatting for the delivery address and the return address on the envelope is different from what it is when we mail it to the future.

The cost of postage is ridiculous.

Most mail trucks aren't even outfitted with any sort of device to travel back in time.

Even if you addressed it perfectly, slapped on an H.G. Wells stamp, and sent it on a time-traveling mail truck, your letter would still land in the wrong slot—moments before some vandal raided the box for pension checks meant for the old guy who never stops yelling at you to get off his lawn.

Mom wrote a letter to herself once.

She typed it up, put some postage on it, and mailed it to herself a few days in the future.

I've often wondered if there was a way to communicate with my past-self, what would I say.

Would I reveal the future to my past-self, or just keep everything hush-hush?

There are plenty of time-traveling stories out there which explore this premise, and as such, I'm not going to subject you to my own efforts on the matter.

At best, there will be a bunch of jumping back and forth to different points in time. Such a device in a story like this will work like the MacGuffin rug that was inappropriately removed from the apartment of the wrong Lebowski.

"That rug really tied the room together."

Snapshots of the different points in my life won't be the only thing you'll see in the pattern in the rug though. Included is a healthy mix of pop culture references—some direct, some subtle—that those of us in Generation X have carried with us since the days of feathered hair and calculating the shrinkage risk of our 501s after their first wash. To round everything out, there will be several confusing assaults on the native tongue.

Just know that most of it is on purpose.

It should also be stated right here and now that the bulk of what you are about to read really happened, no matter how far-fetched it seems.

For the parts which seem to be a little outlandish to have ever happened, feel free to assume that I completely made it up. Your assumption wouldn't be too far off the mark.

Please enjoy.

Prologue

<u>Five Years Ago</u>

"Guess what?"

"Chicken butt."

"Huh?"

Yeah, I didn't really expect Mom to get that joke, but I played that card anyway.

"Nothing. What's up?"

"I bought a new car."

"No kidding. What'd you get?" She told me. What perfect timing. I had seen a meme or a joke somewhere recently, and I was about to engineer a full out re-enactment of that witty little play on words. I asked her if they had a certain restaurant up there in Colorado where she lived.

"Yes, we do. Why?"

"I need you to get a friend and a camera and go take a picture."

<u>Present Day</u>

It's ten minutes after five and we're waiting for dinner in the spacious dining room of Los Prados Verdes Center for Nursing & Rehabilitation.

Country music is being piped into the speakers overhead. The station plays nothing from the current century. That's a good thing, as no one in the room is from the current century either. Although I never really considered myself a fan of the genre, I'm continually amazed at just how much of it I know.

The kitchen commandos have brought out two push carts with about fifteen trays. The nursing staff will start passing them out to the residents who have been placed strategically throughout the dining room.

Linda is the only resident who isn't seated in a wheelchair. Everyone else is, including Mom.

"COFFEE! WITH CREAM AND SUGAR!" Mr. Wilson is seated at the back end of the dining room facing a large bay window. Just a few minutes ago he had barked an order at one of the window attendants to open the curtains. He wanted to see the roller coaster at the amusement park on the other side of the highway.

For what it's worth, there are no window attendants to attend to Mr. Wilson's request.

Linda and Gwendolyn break their own conversation about the questionable treatment they're getting to respond to Mr. Wilson's demands. "There's no one here to give you coffee yet." It's a foregone conclusion that on that fateful day when the residents start rioting, it will be based on the battle plans that those two have drawn up.

Ellen, who's at the other end of the dining room and a little closer to us responds. "I'd like some coffee." She addresses the lady sitting at the table with her. "Would you?"

Pour myself a cup of ambition

And yawn and stretch and try to come to life

Tio Hector, his sharply dressed nephews, and their Ouija Board are nowhere to be found. This is a relief. The minute the good people at Los Prados Verdes Center for Nursing & Rehabilitation take that guy and his desk bell on as a resident, I'm getting Mom out of there.

Mr. OK and the female version of Doc Brown are seated at a table together. Doc Brown sports a post-combustion flash of white hair and the ability to talk endlessly about gigawatts and a variety of other subjects at 88 miles an hour. She reminds me of a character I saw in a movie once.

Rest assured; I've seen that movie more than once.

Doc Brown's dining partner just stares at her over the top of his glasses and periodically says "**OKAAAY.**" in his loud, yet strained voice.

Minnie and Rosa are stationed close by. Minnie doesn't talk much, but Rosa is carrying on a conversation in Spanish which I can only hope is as intriguing as the one-sided discussion Doc Brown and Mr. OK are having.

"**OKAAAY.**"

If only my Spanish was more colloquial and conversational. Sure I can conjugate a verb and order from a menu, but I want to know *porque el bano esta cerrado,* and why it matters to Rosa so much.

Linda and Gwendolyn start talking about the local races in the upcoming election. "Biden is the president right now," announces one of the nurses. "He's more confused than all of you put together!"

"COFFEE! CREAM AND SUGAR!"

"*...como mantequilla en el chango pelon....*"

"Are we going to eat supper?"

I paused my attention to the ambient conversation and turn to the reason I'm here. "Hey Mom, this stuff is better than all of those cheesy made-for-TV movies you get to watch every day."

Verbally, Mom is non-responsive, but that roll of her eyes tells me that she's still aware of her surroundings. *I cannot believe that I've been planted here in a nursing home doing nothing but watching TV all day! Is this what the rest of my life is going to look like?*

Something smells good, but not so good that my stomach growls in anticipation. After all, I won't be eating until later when I get home. Dinner is for Mom and the other residents.

"I'm going home tomorrow." Ellen announces. She's not. "Do you want to come with me?" She asks Minnie, who just glares at her.

Minnie has shot me a glare or two, however to this point, the only non-verbal discussions I fully understand come from Mom.

I've been trying to get Minnie to warm up to me lately just by waving or saying "Hi" to her. She still looks at me with disdain. When the riots start, she'll pledge fealty to the chief insurrectionists (Linda and Gwendolyn) and then proceed to keep everyone in line with an iron fist. I'm fairly sure I'll be one of the first ones up against the wall, and I don't even work there.

Barely getting' by, it's all takin' and no givin'

They just use your mind and they never give you credit

Dinner arrives. There's a ticket on the tray which lists Mom's name and the menu items which have been pureed and plopped lovingly on the plate for her consumption. At the bottom of the ticket, in bold capital letters is the word "FEEEDER". I guess the 'E' key was stuck that day when the meal tickets were being printed.

This is a signal to those who care for Mom that she's unable to feed herself. There are a few other residents in the dining room who have the same issue. They're usually seated together so one nurse can feeed two residents at a time.

Dinner is the pureed version of the worst kitchen table memories from my youth, all consolidated into a brown casserole dish with a glass lid. It's called meatloaf, and knowing what it is has changed my opinion on the aroma. I proceed to feed it to Mom while hiding my contempt for the unfortunate menu option and my glee for not having to eat it.

This stuff isn't as good as the meatloaf I used to make.

Quit making that face over it Randy. You used to eat it all the time.

—A, it smells bad, and 2, I'm pretty sure I ate it under duress. I haven't had that stuff since I was a teenager.

The only thing that is more disturbing is that dress you're wearing.

What's wrong with it?

—It's not yours or anything you would ever wear. The colors and patterns on it, much like this meatloaf, make me long for the euphoria I get from vertigo and food poisoning.

So how did I get it?

—I don't know. Somebody put it on you one day and decided it was yours.

Thirty minutes later, there are only a few residents left in the dining room who haven't finished the evening's vittles.

> *Like grandma and grandpa used to play*

> *Then I'll float on down the river*

"Hey Mom, there's a song we know. We saw them a few times back in the 80s." A flash of recognition goes across Mom's face as it occurs to me that a shirt I got at one of those concerts is now in a storage bin in my garage.

Ellen backs away from her table to make a run for it. A member of staff notices this and calls out to the would-be escapee before she can get too far. "Ellen, you need to eat some more."

"I KNOW!" Ellen is usually compliant and an all-around sweetheart, but that response sounded a little indignant. One of the C.N.A.'s approaches Ellen with an appeal for her low blood sugar.

> *Play some back-home, come-on music*

> *That comes from the heart*

"I don't know where I got the bubble bath."

I offer another spoonful to Mom, who refuses it. *Get that out of my face!*

By now she's eaten about 80% of her meal. This is good compared to what it was six months ago. "Ok, let's move on to some dessert. Looks like some chocolatey goodness in there."

There's a fine line between a pureed brownie and brownie batter.

Members of the nursing staff gradually remove each of the residents from of the dining room, leaving us by ourselves.

> *Then I'll float on down the river*
>
> *To a Cajun hideaway*

We get through about half of the chocolatey goodness and Mom signals that she's done. That's fine.

I've had a long day, and I'm done too. I wonder if I've signaled that.

I put my mask back on in accordance with some arbitrary policy about whether one can catch or spread a virus based on whether they're seated in a dining room or walking down a hallway, and I begin to wheel Mom back to her room.

Halfway between the dining room and Mom's room we encounter the nurses station. Most of the other wheelchair-bound residents who were in that dining room with us are now set up in a circle around that station. The nurses tend to leave the residents at this staging ground before and after meals for a variety of reasons. Some of them are making a connection to their next activity involving mixed martial arts and bingo. Others are waiting for movie night in the café which is just off to the side of the nurses station. According to the activity calendar, the movie is residents' choice.

I wonder if *Cocoon* is on the list of choices.

Several of the residents just sit there in their wheelchairs performing a supervisory role over the nurses. Deep down, I know they're gathering intelligence and studying patterns in preparation for the riots to come. Minnie breaks her concentration on the nurses' activities to glare at me as I walk by.

I crack a smile from behind my mask. She's underwhelmed.

A few weeks ago, I encountered Mom sitting in the same round with a few other residents. They were gathering reconnaissance. The look on her face reminded me of those times in my youth when my poorly executed chore work failed to live up to her standards. All these years later I wondered if that look was being used as non-verbal signals to her geriatric comrades and the rumors of insurrection I kept hearing about.

We carefully navigate the obstacle course of wheelchairs and their cargo and then break free in an open-field run down the hallway where Mom's room is.

We encounter Martin in the hallway on the way. No staring or glaring from Martin, mind you. He always asks how I'm doing and tells me it's good to see me. Sometimes there's a handshake or a fist bump.

Mom's room is in the same condition it was when we left. The lights are dimmed, the bed is made with her owl blanket on top, and the TV is playing another Christmas movie. That TV has been on the same channel all week.

I honestly didn't realize that girl from that 80s sitcom, the real-life little sister of what's-his-face from that other 80s sitcom, had done so many of these movies.

I wheel Mom in, and park her between the bed and the recliner facing the TV. She's never been a fan of TV, but it keeps her attention now.

"Okay Mom, I need to get going."

There's that look again.

Everyone knows that look they get from their mother. It's the look that tells you that you've just perpetrated more than a minor indiscretion, and continued behavior in the same manner is going to result in unpleasant consequences. You have to the count of three to correct your behavior, and you've already chalked up one on the board. My youth was peppered with such admonishments.

That's one.

At least that's what that look used to mean. Nowadays, it's a manifestation of her trying to process the fact that I was leaving for the night. I get it every time I ask her a multiple-choice question or announce that I'm leaving.

I rubbed her shoulders and expressed my love for her and told her good night.

"Good night." Sometimes she responds, sometimes she doesn't.

You aren't going to make me watch this stupid movie again, are you? Can you at least change the channel?

Randy?

I stepped out of her room and pulled her door to a more closed position. Being at the end of a main hallway, I'd rather not have every passerby be able to peek in and check out which Christmas movie she's watching.

Two of the nurses are in the hallway doing whatever it is that nurses at long term care facilities do whenever they're not getting Mom out of bed, dressed and into the wheelchair, out of the wheelchair, undressed, and back into bed. We exchange pleasantries and I head out.

There was a time just a few months ago when leaving Mom like this would generate feelings of devastation, guilt, and general lousiness. Those feelings subsided when I came to terms with the fact that I did the right thing by getting her into this place.

Mom doesn't have the ability to share her backstory with the nurses, doctors, therapists, and other members of staff who are charged with her well-being. Since I'm not always there to share Mom's origin story, I've put a picture of Mom on display in her room which tells a story. When others see that picture, they get a hint of what things used to be like.

The woman in that picture never sat around watching TV all day. She hated TV and assigned the ills of society to it many times in my youth.

Instead, the woman in that picture went out and did stuff. She lived in the valley of Pikes Peak and liked to hike around what she referred to as "yonder hill". She loved "yonder hill" and even named her business (her encore career) after it.

The woman in that picture had a sense of humor and a sarcastic streak that periodically continues to reveal itself.

When I entered her room the other day and asked her what she was up to, she surprised me twice. The first surprise was that she responded, and the second surprise was that she used sarcasm.

"About 5'4".

That made my day.

She told the story for years that she got those attributes from me.

Whisking Mom away from the land of "yonder hill" in favor of getting her the proper attention and care she needed was tricky enough.

I'll never know whether Mom was coincidently scheduled for mental and physical collapse at just the time I arrived to save her, or if the mere fact of saving her brought on the decline.

I'm not going to burn calories on trying to figure that one out.

Even still, the thought of telling the story about getting Mom from Colorado to Texas with its multi-layered cacophony of plot lines never occurred to me until I found myself watching a separate multi-layered cacophony of plot lines happening all at once in the middle of the dining room at Los Prados Verdes Center for Nursing & Rehabilitation last November.

If I were to give you the two-minute elevator speech on how Mom came to be in my care, I would tell you that last July on a Friday, I showed up at her door in Colorado and said, "Let's go." By brunch time on Saturday, we had packed up her car and took a one-way road trip to Texas where she would come live with me.

Getting Mom out of Colorado was that quick. There was no time to contact friends or the rest of her community to say "Goodbye".

Shortly after arriving here in Texas, Mom's health went into a rapid decline which required us to seek additional care for her at Los Prados Verdes Center for Nursing & Rehabilitation.

When Mom told me about her new car all those years ago, she jumped at the chance to follow through with my picture suggestion. It never occurred to either of us back then that I would use that picture to tell her story.

Five years ago, Mom and a friend drove to a steakhouse which is part of a nationwide chain and parked in the back. While Mom stayed in the car, her friend got out, produced a camera, and framed a picture of Mom sitting in her new car with that steakhouse in the background.

I had that picture printed, framed, and labeled so that it could be put on prominent display in room 209 in Los Prados Verdes Center for Nursing & Rehabilitation where Mom resides today.

The picture features Barb, out back the Outback in her Outback.

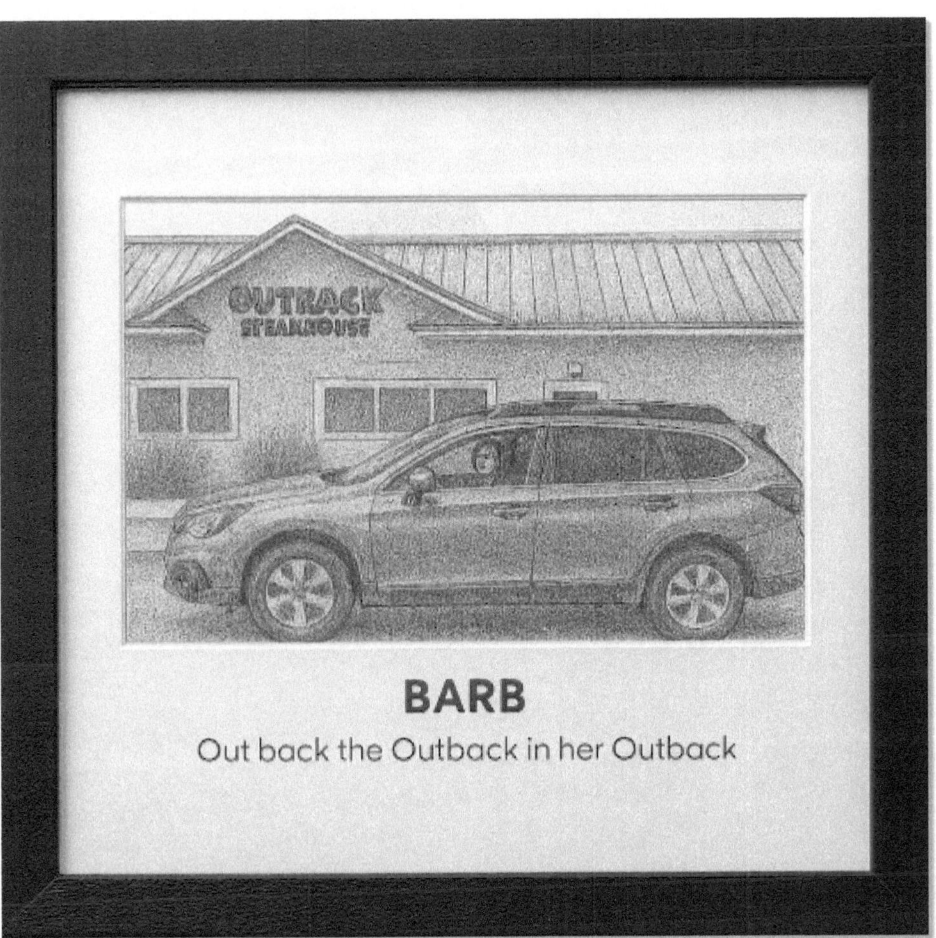

BARB

Out back the Outback in her Outback

Dear Barb

January 19, 2016

Dear Barb,

After your lifetime of challenges - everyone has them - I love who you have become today. You're outgoing, and eager to help others. And you're no longer living in fear of rejection and/or judgment!

Yesterday, you reached 4 years of Lifetime status in Weight Watchers! As if that weren't enough, you've also committed to weekly exercise with a trainer, which has been happening for 18 months now! Good job!

You've come so far since you quit working in corporate America! I truly love who you are today and look forward to many more years of your contribution to society!

Not only are you joyfully using Emotion Code and Body Code, to bring all types of healing to others, but you're also volunteering your time to a homeless dog shelter, by doing their accounting. And you're an occasional volunteer at the hospital, as well. That you were able to do that, after leaving under less than desirable circumstances, speaks worlds about your ability to forgive!

Volunteering at the church will be coming soon, too, just as soon as that can be arranged. And doing Emotion Code and Body Code for anyone attending there will certainly help many more than you are currently reaching.

I truly love the new you, Barb! Keep up the good work and continue working to extend your reach to the world!

Love,

Barb

Too Many Ooga-Chakas

Ooga-Chaka, Ooga-Ooga,

Ooga-Chaka, Ooga-Ooga,

Ooga-Chaka, Ooga-Ooga

"Hooked on a Feeling" is a 1968 pop song written by Mark James and originally performed by B.J. Thomas. I was today-years old when I took to the internet and learned that little tidbit from the first result by my search engine of choice.

Going further, I didn't know B.J. Thomas had sung that song, but I did know that he sang the theme song from that one sitcom back in the 80s which featured the big brother of that girl that was in that other sitcom that was now doing all those Christmas movies on the single channel perpetually broadcasted onto Mom's TV.

I'm more familiar with the 1974 version of "Hooked on a Feeling" by Blue Swede in which the "Ooga-Chaka" was not in the original version with B.J. Thomas singing. The inspiration from that chant came from an ongoing chant in the 1959 song "*Running Bear*" by Johnny Preston.

Many years ago, I took a snippet of that chant from the Blue Swede version of "Hooked on a Feeling" and made it the ringtone on my phone. I always found the chant to be like the noise my phlegmatic washing machine makes when the spin cycle can't negotiate my vast collection of dark solids and plaid unmentionables.

Someone was calling, and the ringtone told me it wasn't anyone in my immediate circle who warranted a customized tone.

I had loosened up the controls on my phone recently to allow more callers to trigger that chant. I had decided to take unknown calls in case they were about Mom, and not those who were trying to sell me insurance benefits, travel packages, solar panels, debt relief, or extended vehicle warranties.

Instead, the people who made my phone chant were calling to express their concerns about Mom. That's what happens when you're listed as an emergency contact for others. Unknown people contact you with stories about how your loved one ran out of gas on some highway or had challenges parking her low-mileage, 2011 Subaru Outback in her designated parking spot just out back of apartment H at the Enchanted Springs Apartment Complex.

Granted, calls like this weren't the harbinger of Mom's condition. They were just more signals that I may need to step in sooner rather than later for the management of Mom's life.

My concerns went into high gear in April when I called Mom to make arrangements for her to fly to Texas in May when my new grandson was due to arrive.

Up until then, calls with Mom in the previous months had been a little troubling when she would talk about having a bad memory. I had always known her to have an incredibly good one.

In fact it was so good that I had to develop some impressive skills in my youth if I was going to slip a lie or two past her ever watchful eye.

I had a few frustrating calls with her at the beginning of the year because of technical issues she was having with her laptop. Walking her through those issues and even loading the program which would allow me to take control of her PC turned into a couple of heated conversations. "I'm sorry for getting frustrated and losing my patience Mom. It's just that we've done this several times before with no issue and now we can't even get a screen share program loaded for you."

My concerns got to a point where I offered to set her up with a long-term care insurance policy during the new year. The first policy we looked at went nowhere because she refused to see a doctor to qualify her for the coverage. Mom has been an ardent detractor of western medicine for years. She wasn't about to see a doctor.

When we submitted the application for the second choice in policies, the underwriter required a mental health evaluation where someone would visit Mom for an interview and skedaddle right on out of there with no physical exam. Mom was amenable to that, so we moved forward.

A few weeks later, the agent we were working with called to let me know that Mom had failed the evaluation for reasons unknown.

Looking back, I'm guessing the person who conducted the interview could see the future.

In the end, we settled on a supplemental policy that technically isn't to be considered a long-term care policy. A month later, Mom called me to advise that she was taking a memory boosting supplement and wasn't experiencing the memory issues she had before. I had her blessing to cancel the policy.

I politely declined.

When I called her in April to arrange for her to fly to Texas to meet her great grandson, I could tell that something was wrong. I couldn't keep her focused on finding time in May to fly into Dallas where the kid would arrive.

Mom was focused on her aging cocker spaniel Brandi, and what to do about her while she was away. Her dog sitter had limited availability at the end of May, and Brandi couldn't just be boarded with the vet.

Understandable.

She then told me that several strangers had been in and out of her apartment for the last few weeks.

She told me that she hadn't filed her taxes yet, which meant she was already a week or two late.

She told me the only thing she was eating was mint chocolate chip ice cream.

Nothing else.

She told me about her friend Cheryl who had expressed similar concerns about Mom.

What had started out as a single task phone call to book a flight for Mom turned into a multi-faceted checklist.

I still had to get a flight booked, but the dates were up in the air.

I told her I would do her taxes and needed her to send her paperwork.

I had to find out what was in the memory boost supplement that was messing with her cognitive abilities.

I had to make contact with Cheryl for an independent assessment. Fortunately, I had the presence of mind to ask Mom for contact information for Cheryl, and she provided it.

Within ten minutes of ending that call, I called Thumper to share my concerns.

Right around the time he entered junior high, my kid brother had a collection of habits that irritated Mom to no end. "Stop swaying in the breeze!" was a common admonishment she would deliver on a regular basis. I guess watching him tilt back and forth like that gave her the sense that he was rocking the forest.

But it wasn't swaying in the breeze that got him the nickname of Thumper.

Instead, it was the way he constantly tapped his feet. Someone at school gave him that name and it stuck.

Thumper and I never speak on the phone. Instead we text each other. After all, it's the 21st century, and what are a couple of middle-aged men in their 50's going to 'talk' about?

For me to call him was an unprecedented move.

On that call, I outlined everything that had just taken place on the earlier call with Mom. We agreed that Mom would get a call from her other favorite son that night. I then went to bed but did not go to sleep. A full night's sleep would elude me until July 14th when my worries about Mom being alone were assuaged.

In the interim, I was able to reach out to Cheryl and get confirmation of my concerns. Sleep continued to be elusive in the meantime.

We eventually booked a flight for Mom to fly into Dallas during Memorial Day week. This was a matter of days after the expected arrival of my grandson and coincided with birthdays that Mom and I would have in the first few days of June. There were issues with getting care for Brandi during that week, so we rebooked for a flight to take place on Labor Day.

"I don't think she's going to make it to Labor Day." Cheryl lamented to me on a call in June.

A few days after my grandson was born, I was sitting in an Air BnB somewhere in Dallas. It was my birthday.

The new kid and his parents had come over for a visit. His poor mom had been physically wrecked that previous Friday in the birthing process, so she was pretty worn out.

Mom called to touch base on some tax documents she had found which would help me do her taxes for her. I spent the next hour unsuccessfully walking her through the process of taking a picture of the documents and sending them to me.

In that whole time, she never mentioned my birthday.

Over the next few weeks, I lost contact with Mom.

She wouldn't or couldn't answer the phone.

She didn't respond to my texts or my emails.

At one point Cheryl dropped by Mom's apartment and figured out that Mom was not charging her phone.

Even when the phone did get charged, Mom was still not responding to any of my calls, texts, or emails.

Having determined that her phone was too complicated for her, I did the next best thing. I bought her a phone. I added contact information for me, my wife, and my brother to that phone. I printed instructions on how to use the phone to call me. I then shipped it to her.

Ooga-Chaka, Ooga-Ooga,

Ooga-Chaka, Ooga-Ooga,

Ooga-Chaka, Ooga-Ooga

I looked at the chanting phone hoping that Mom was calling me from her new phone.

It wasn't her. Instead, her friend Cheryl was calling.

"Hello?"

"Hi." It wasn't Cheryl.

"Hi Mom." Mom was calling from Cheryl's phone. "How are you?"

"Brandi died."

Mom had just lost the last reason to keep things together.

She was still eating ice cream and nothing else.

She didn't care about her taxes, and I was guessing her finances may have been in peril too. She gave me that hint last month in a text message advising that she had been evicted. She explained it away as a misunderstanding with the management team of the Enchanted Springs Apartment Complex where she lived. It turns out the lease for her space in apartment H was up and the property manager had delicately told her that she should consider other living arrangements.

We all knew that Brandi was Mom's last motivation to do anything. She no longer had a reason to get up every day and participate in life. No one was relying on her to provide food, water, or a walk.

Brandi had been gone for a few days, and Mom had done nothing about it. She hadn't told anyone, nor had she tried to take Brandi's body to be cremated as planned. It was fortunate that Cheryl showed up at her door when she did.

A plan was put into action for Cheryl and Mom to take Brandi to a vet the next day to have her cremated.

Here in Texas, it was go-time.

I hadn't formulated any type of plan which was littered with a whole bunch of if/then statements. Sleep continued to elude me as I lie awake that night mapping things out.

I was going to fly to Colorado the next week and then drive back to Texas in a low-mileage 2011 Outback, with Mom seated comfortably in the passenger seat, or bound and gagged in the cargo hold.

From Apartment H To Room 209

A Prelude To A Series Of Delays

Thursday morning took forever to get here.

Everything I had worried about for the last several months, all the planning I had done in the last week, and all the rehearsed speeches were now converging into a conversation I would have with Mom in a matter of hours.

She didn't know when I would arrive because I didn't want her to drive to the airport to pick me up.

To say that my plans for that day were fluid and flexible was an understatement. It's rare that I go anywhere and not have a detailed plan for achieving my objective.

All I had to do was get on a plane in San Antonio, connect in Dallas to another plane bound for the Rocky Mountains, score a ride to apartment H where Mom would be, convince her to return with me, and drive back to Texas in a low-mileage, 2011 Subaru Outback with Mom either comfortably seated in the passenger seat, or bound and gagged in the cargo hold with the luggage.

In the end, it worked out that I wouldn't be allowed to keep a strict itinerary.

It started Thursday morning with me sitting at the gate, waiting to board the plane that wasn't there yet.

Okay fine, if this is the worstest thing that will happen on this trip, that's great. Let's get it out of the way.

I'll pause a moment to reflect on my misplaced optimism.

A few hours later I was sitting in the plane as it was preparing to leave San Antonio.

The delay festered. Everyone was on the plane, and the doors were closed. Some of us who had places to be and things to do were buckled in with our tray table up and our seats in an upright position so that we could take off to that destination a few hundred miles north so that we could make our connecting flight for destinations even further north.

The rest of the heathens were reclined and occupied in slapdash, devil-may-care activities on their personal phones and tablets which were looked upon by the FAA as non-conducive to safe and successful air travel.

A voice came over the intercom. It was the captain speaking, using the same voice every airplane captain uses to inform you that other forces have wrestled control of your destiny from your white knuckled grasp.

There was something about weather between San Antonio and Dallas that would require that we swing out west over Abilene instead of taking a direct flight.

There was additional information about getting more fuel so that we could swing out west over Abilene. It seems the pump jockeys charged with giving us gas misunderstood the number of gallons that were needed and put way too much in. That was intolerable to the captain, who subsequently had to go outside and expedite the removal of the excess fuel.

To this day, I don't know if they were out there taking turns sucking on the syphon. My carefully selected aisle seat didn't afford me a view of the gas cap.

In the meantime, I got the impression that I was the only one in steerage fully invested in a full-on mental breakdown at the premise that the airline industry had taken indecent liberties with their customers in recent years. Granted, the weather issue and the misplacement of a comma or two in the calculation of gallons of fuel it took to swing west over Abilene magnified my anxiety about what I had to do that day.

So I sat there, belted in with my tray table locked in place and my seat in an upright position chanting "Serenity Now".

A message appeared on my phone from the airline app. I was going to miss my connection and needed to reschedule.

Of course.

Even worserer, there were no more flights for Thursday. I wouldn't get to Mom until Friday.

Did I mention Abilene?

Grandma, the mother of the focus of today's mission, had lived in Abilene for several years. Whenever I hear "Abilene", I think of Grandma. I can trace my organizational skills, my need for a plan, and my pedantries back to Grandma via her only child, my Mom.

Grandma and Mom had a strained relationship. The downstream impacts of that strained relationship were omnipresent throughout my life until Grandma passed away in 1995. I'm pretty sure the last time Grandma and Mom spoke was shortly after Grandpa passed in 1993.

I'm not aware of whether they ever reconciled their differences. Even today, thirty years after Grandma's passing, I make it a point not to even mention her to Mom.

Nonetheless, the premise of swinging out over Abilene on the endeavor to rescue Mom invigorated the perpetual flux of my pyloric valve. Of course I came by that honestly. Mom's valve was always snapping open and shut whenever Grandma's presence was imminent.

I texted Mom telling her my flight was delayed and that I would be there tomorrow. Arrival details to follow.

I would have to make arrangements to spend the night in *scoff* Dallas.

I hate that place.

Sure I have family there, but otherwise I hate it.

It goes back to the days when watching professional football and basketball was an exercise in sports entertainment, free of political statements.

Irregardlessly, I would have to stay there on Thursday night.

So the loosely scheduled Thursday mission to board a plane in San Antonio, connect in Dallas, land in Colorado Springs, knock on Mom's door and convince her to return to Texas with me had changed to a multi-day event.

Fortunately, my brother was in Dallas to put me up for the night, but not without including me in some behavior of his which had inappropriately been deemed to be inappropriate, even though in the grand scheme of things, was perfectly appropriate.

<u>Thursdays With Thumper</u>

For what seemed to be days, if not weeks, I sat there in the middle seat of an aisle nestled in steerage, trying to make my way from Texas to somewhere in the Rocky Mountains to see Mom.

I was done.

I was done with the tight quarters.

I was done with that kid to my right looking out the window, minding his own business and not being a burden to the other two occupants of the aisle.

I was done with that chicken lunch which had been served shortly after take-off.

I was done with the disembodied, dulcet-toned voice of the captain admonishing us to buckle up because we were now on what would be a bumpy approach to our destination.

I was done with the side effects of "a little bumpy" which had suddenly manifested in the pyloric valve.

I was done with the clammy skin and shortness of breath.

I was done with that kid next to me not giving me a good excuse to lash out at him.

I checked out the window to see how close we were to the ground, hoping that the person flying this plane didn't have the fish.

We weren't far, but we weren't close enough.

I was feeling lousy, and something was about to happen.

Where's that barf bag?

I rifled through the pocket of the seat in front of me looking for a vessel to receive a soon to be rejected chicken lunch.

Moments later, things were better.

Kind of.

I was no longer wedged between two people and unable to move. I was now out of that aisle, off the plane and swearing off air travel for the rest of my life. At the same time, I was making my way to the terminal with a newly presented mission to accomplish as quickly and discreetly possible.

The first thing I encountered was a crowd of people welcoming a soldier or two who were home from deployment.

If the soldiers had committed the same atrocity I just did, the remnants of bile would have blended nicely with the camouflage in their duds. I didn't have the convenience of camouflage attire to hide my most recent indiscretion.

"Did you barf?" There was Mom at the gate, dispensing with any discretion over the indiscretion I had hoped to hide.

Never mind the fact that I had just waded through a herd of patriotic well-wishers while I was trying to conceal the contents of an upchucked chicken lunch on my shirt.

Never mind the fact that the kid sitting in the window seat next to me had received the brunt of my gastronomical mischief on his left pant leg and was now in close enough proximity to hear the inquiry.

Mom was there to greet me—and my shirt stain—and immediately assessed how my flight had gone.

"Sshhh." I admonished her in a hushed tone. "I threw up on that kid right over there."

"Oh."

"If you'll just hang tight here for a minute, I'm going to go clean up."

I left Mom to stand there with my backpack and went to the restroom where I encountered that kid. "Hey, I'm really sorry about that. The turbulence got me pretty quickly there." That wasn't the first time I had uttered that statement to that kid.

He finished wiping his pant leg off and looked at me. "Okay."

Well what else are you supposed to say when an older person does that to you on the plane?

That was 1991.

The only concern any of us had about cognitive decline was not in Mom, but in my Grandfather. At the time, Grandma was seeking out a nursing home in Abilene which could take care of him.

Thirty-something years later, on a Thursday afternoon, I got off a plane in Dallas.

There was no vomit on my shirt, or on the pant leg of the person who was sitting next to me. Credit for that goes to the 30-year-old policy about not eating on an airplane. That policy has allowed me to live a life free of surprise regurgitations.

Swearing off air travel has been more difficult.

I had missed my connection to Colorado Springs that day due to weather and other airline-borne delays.

When I received word in San Antonio that I would miss my connection, I was able to get on another flight out of Dallas early on Friday morning. I would be spending the night with Thumper who had an apartment downtown.

"There's an issue with my truck." He texted me while I was making my way to the pick-up zone at the airport in Dallas. "You'll need to get a ride to my apartment."

I'll take this moment to summarize the progress of the trip so far and add some tangential context.

My flight out of San Antonio was delayed, and we had to swing out over Abilene to get to Dallas. That's like swinging out over the Mississippi River to fly from Florida to New York.

Because of the delay leaving San Antonio, I had missed my connecting flight in Dallas and had to reschedule it to Friday morning.

I would be spending the night with my brother Thumper in an apartment complex downtown. There is a bar within the same complex.

Patrons of the bar tend to park in the parking garage for the apartment in spots which are reserved for tenants of the apartment complex. The apartment management actively has vehicles which have been deemed to be inappropriately parked in that garage towed and impounded in some city-run lot stationed light years away.

Thumper had been in a wreck recently and was driving a rental.

Management at the apartment didn't recognize Thumper's rental which was appropriately parked. They subsequently deemed the vehicle to be inappropriately parked and had it towed to the city-run lot stationed light years away.

It should be noted here that my intention was to bring Mom through Dallas on the trip back to San Antonio to spend the night. The thought that the low-mileage, 2011 Subaru Outback we would be driving could potentially be deemed to be inappropriately parked and subsequently towed and impounded in some city-run lot stationed light years away was a little disconcerting.

When I return to Dallas with Mom seated comfortably in the passenger seat or bound and gagged in the cargo hold of her low-mileage, 2011 Subaru Outback the next day, I may have to park the Outback out back the Outback down the street.

So the next step in this quest to bring Mom to Texas began as my first Uber ride deposited me at the apartment complex which featured a bar. A little later, Thumper and I subsequently had to flag down another Uber driver in a rented Tesla so that we could be taken to some city-run lot stationed light years away to reacquire the rental which had been inappropriately deemed to have been inappropriately parked.

Have you ever tried to get a rental that you barely recognize out of impound?

Have you ever tried to show proof of ownership or insurance under such circumstances?

Have you ever tried to convince the attendant at some city-run lot stationed light years away that the rental you were driving which had inappropriately been deemed to have been inappropriately parked that you weren't the one who would be paying for the towing and impound fees, and that said fees would be paid by the outfit which had inappropriately deemed the rental to have been inappropriately parked?

My misplaced optimism was soaring. Everything that could have gone wrong on this adventure was being dispatched upfront. Once I got out of Dallas, everything would be fine and smooth sailing.

I'll pause to reflect on that.

An hour later, we had made our way back downtown in the rental which had been inappropriately impounded. We were now going to a cantina for dinner. Maybe we could find a pilot to get us to Alderaan while we were there.

"Is it me, or does she smell like rainbows?"

"Funny you should mention that." I responded. "I started writing something a few years ago where..."

"And did you see those blue eyes?" Our server / bartender was a beautiful young thing of Asian descent who had become the focus of Thumper's attention in recent months.

"Yup. They're contacts." I responded.

"See, now how do you know that? Someone else told me the same thing."

"Because when you put blue tinted contacts on brown eyes, that's the color you get."

"Well why didn't I know that?"

"Good question. Why didn't you? You're 50-somethin'. You should've gotten a clue by now." It's always good to see my brother and shoot the bull over the stupidest little thing. Even still, the stupidest little thing wasn't on my mind at the time.

"So how are you going to get Mom to come back with you?"

I halted my decision process between the flautas and the enchiladas and looked at him. "I don't know. It's between asking her to come, demanding that she come, or tricking her to come."

He looked at me and processed each of those approaches but couldn't immediately offer a solution. We had an unspoken discussion about how Mom wasn't easy to trick in our formative years. We silently and mutually recalled how each of our respective stubborn streaks were impressive and born from her. Making demands wouldn't work. Furthermore, we didn't have to utter the words that she didn't really want to return to Texas, so a simple request could be met with resistance.

"Yeah."

"Yup."

She Was Gone When I Got There

Friday morning arrived in a different way for me than it ever had.

I woke up on a sectional couch in a downtown Dallas apartment, and Thumper's dog wasn't happy with my presence.

On top of the limited quality and quantity of sleep I got that night (nothing new as of late), I was also sore from sleeping on a sectional couch in a downtown Dallas apartment where the dog wasn't very happy about it. I had already accepted that it would only be a few more days before I could get some quality sleep, back in my own bed, with Mom safely installed in the spare bedroom.

Less than an hour later, Thumper was depositing me at the passenger drop-off zone at DFW. No matter the airport, I'm always reminded of that scene from Airplane! where the disembodied voices carry on an argument about which zone is for loading and unloading of passengers. As I opened the door to get out of the truck, Thumper offered up some words of encouragement.

"I just want to tell you both good luck. We're all counting on you."

"Thanks. If all goes well, I'll be knocking on your door tomorrow night with Mom either seated comfortably in the passenger seat or bound and gagged in the cargo hold of her low-mileage 2011 Subaru Outback."

"Do you need some duck-tape?"

"Duck-tape?"

"Duck, duct, take your pick."

The next thing I know, I'm on the plane in a window seat. An elderly lady sits next to me in the much-maligned middle seat, and her daughter who I estimated to be only a few years older than me was on the aisle. She produced a tablet and set it up on the tray in front of her mother. She punched in an access code, pulled up a streaming service, and selected a movie for mom to watch on the flight to Colorado Springs.

My hard and fast rule about eating on airplanes came to mind.

Upchucking a chicken lunch on an airplane while sitting next to an elderly lady who appears to be in her own state of cognitive decline is not something you want to do nowadays. The saving grace I had with that event thirty years ago was the refreshing lack of cell phones, the internet, and instant fame for our occasional lack of dignity and grace.

I wondered if selecting movies for Mom to watch would be among the activities I would be relegated to once I had custody of her.

Looking back on that moment, I wish that were the only thing I had to do.

A few hours later we were on the ground. That impatient little monster in my head was going nuts, but not so much that he was calling for a surprise regurgitation of the contents of my stomach. I had to get off the plane and off to apartment H of the Enchanted Springs Apartment Complex so that I could rescue Mom from whatever imminent danger she was in.

That little monster was going to have to wait for the crowd of people who stood in the aisle, and the elderly lady and her daughter to my immediate right.

So I waited there patiently while a tantrum ensued in the confines of my skull.

The lady turned to me. "Are you in a hurry?" The look on her face told me this woman was a sweetheart. Maybe she wasn't in cognitive decline. For that matter, maybe Mom wasn't either.

Maybe my confirmation bias was getting the better of me, and I was equating cognitive decline with people of a certain age and their inability to navigate 21st century technology like tablets and cell phones and getting gas and eating more than just mint chocolate chip ice cream.

The lady to my right didn't know the half of just how intense my hurry was. She didn't know about the delayed flight, the last-minute decision to make the flight, or even that I was on a mission for which I didn't know whether I would succeed.

She was only making small talk.

I looked at the crowd of passengers in the aisle and responded with all the respect and congeniality she deserved, flavored with just a bit of snark that she would understand was not directed at her. "Oh, I don't think it matters if I'm in a hurry or not."

She understood and smiled.

By now I was resigned to the fact that this whole trip was going to be one giant obstacle course. I would get through it, one pot-hole at a time.

That was fine.

My whole working life in the cubicle had been an ongoing series of obstacle illusions for the last fifteen years.

My ability to work through them was a transferable skill that could be used to get Mom over a thousand miles away from here.

And then I was outside.

There were no disembodied voices on the outdoor speakers arguing about the white zone versus the yellow zone being for loading or unloading.

The weather was beautiful. It was the middle of July and the temperature in Colorado Springs was in the low 80s, a full 15 degrees cooler than what we have in Texas during that time of year. "Oh this is awesome."

Next task, get to Mom's. I specifically did not tell her when I was arriving because I didn't want her driving to pick me up. Instead, I hailed an Uber.

When Patrick showed up in his Volkswagen Fahrvergnügen, I was immediately struck by his uncanny resemblance to a Somali pirate. "Randy?" he asked.

"Yup. How ya doin' Patrick?" I knew who he was because the Uber app had posted his picture, a picture of his car, and his license plate.

"It's getting hot." Patrick had no idea what hot was.

Thirty minutes later, Patrick dropped me off at the wrong apartment H.

It was still within the Enchanted Springs Apartment Complex, just the wrong building. Maybe I had given the wrong address, maybe he mis-entered it into his navigation. Irregardlessly, it was just another obstacle on the course.

Coincidentally enough, Patrick would give me another ride to the same apartment (the correct one this time) a few weeks later when I went back up to start packing Mom's stuff.

Once I made my way to the correct building, the next obstacle presented itself.

Mom's low-mileage, 2011 Subaru Outback wasn't appropriately parked out back apartment H.

Crud.

Had she gone to the airport to pick me up? I hadn't told her what time I was arriving.

Okay, Mom was not here. I had lost contact with her in recent weeks because she wasn't charging her phone. The phone I had shipped her was scheduled to be delivered later today, so she wouldn't have that one at her disposal yet.

At the same time, she did respond to my text yesterday when I told her my flight had been delayed. Holding out hope that she still had a charged phone at hand, I gave her a call to see where she was.

"Hello?" YES! She answered.

"Howdy. I'm here at your apartment but I don't see your car. Are you at home?"

"No, I went to pick up Brandi's ashes, but they weren't ready yet. I'll be there in a few minutes." The thought that Mom was out there driving on her own made me nervous. If I got my way through this whole mission, that would be the last time she would ever drive.

Spoiler alert.

It was.

I took a seat on the steps up to her apartment and waited.

Would she look different?

Would she remember me?

Could she safely park her car?

It only took her a few minutes to get there, but it felt like hours.

As she pulled her low-mileage, 2011 Subaru Outback into the parking spot, I went downstairs to greet her. There appeared to be a look of confusion on her face. Maybe she was wondering how I got there from the airport. Maybe she wasn't expecting me. I could only guess.

I greeted her at her car and involuntarily proceeded to rush her to get out so that we could go upstairs. I don't know if she perceived that the impatient monster in my head was trying to take over.

When we got inside apartment H, my nose told me everything I needed to know. I knew that Brandi had become incontinent in the last year of her life and had taken to using the great indoors as the great outdoors. The unaddressed messes on the carpet, ten days after the poor dog had passed away, was just another piece of the puzzle that something was terribly wrong with Mom. More of those pieces would present themselves before the day was done.

But now it was time for the big speech. I had spent the last week going over and over in my mind how I was going to make this happen.

There were three approaches I could take.

I could trick her. "Hey, let's go on a road trip to San Antonio. I'd love to introduce you to our new dog Charlie. She would love you. On top of that, you and Faith got along really well last time you were there." Once I got her to San Antonio, I would just make it a permanent vacation for her.

I could make a demand of her. "Look I have a power of attorney document for you, and I need to take control of your life. I need you to return to Texas with me."

I could ask her to come with me. "You know, Brandi is gone now, and I really think you'd like living with us where we have two dogs that would love on you just like Brandi did."

I had gone over those three speeches in my mind for the last week or so, not really knowing which one I was going to use.

But now it was go-time. I hugged her and asked her to sit down while I sat down in the loveseat across from her. In all the years I've spent in the cubicle dealing with internal and external customers, I learned that direct transparency is always the best approach.

So I spilled my guts.

<u>The Picture Cube</u>

"When would you want to leave?"

"I think we should get you packed up tonight and head out tomorrow morning in your car." The thought of leaving so soon at such short notice didn't appear to set too well with Mom, but she didn't really say anything and chose to follow my lead.

Given my propensity for having a plan, I had a list on my phone of the things we absolutely had to do before leaving Colorado Springs.

We started by making a quick stop in the management office for the Enchanted Springs Apartment Complex.

A few months ago, someone from this very office had picked up a phone and punched a series of digits on the keypad which in turn activated the customized ringtone on my phone to make a noise resembling the infernal racket my washing machine makes during the spin cycle.

The mere fact that it was the opening chant used in a 1974 pop song was purely coincidental.

The ensuing conversation I had with a member of that office added to the concerns I was developing about Mom at the time.

In addition to making calls to me about her, the office staff had already engaged Mom in a difficult conversation about the status of her lease and how she should consider other living arrangements. Mom didn't seem to understand it that way and believed it was fine for her to stay.

As we entered the office, greetings and pleasantries were exchanged between Mom and the staff. Mom then clammed up, just like we hadn't planned.

I love an awkward pause just as much as the next person, I just didn't realize that Mom was going to initiate one. Since I was the project coordinator here, it seemed only fitting that now was the time to coordinate this thing.

I introduced myself and let the staff know that we were leaving tomorrow. Furthermore, we were giving notice that Mom was leaving the apartment. I made additional arrangements with them that we would be completely out within 60 days. They were generous and gave us a few extra weeks. This would give me until the end of September to completely vacate.

Afterward, we went to lunch and ate Mongolian barbeque. "Ya know the last time we were in this place was on my birthday three years ago. "Kung Fu Fighting" was playing over the sound system."

I almost asked Mom if she remembered what she gave me that year for my birthday, but I opted not to. If she was having memory issues, I didn't want to stress her out with a pop quiz.

There were points throughout the afternoon where Mom expressed an interest in going to see friends to say goodbye. We just didn't have the time to do that, and I didn't want to allow her to get off task.

The next stop was the bank. Mom had a safe deposit box there which had some heirlooms, old currency, and the original copies of her estate planning documents she had executed a few years ago.

I was a joint owner on Mom's accounts and the safe deposit box, so I would have been able to get that stuff on my own on future trips to pack up her apartment. It was better that I had her there as a willing participant.

The day progressed and the errands which needed to be run had been run.

Now we had to pack.

Fortunately, Mom was willing to come to Texas seated comfortably in the passenger seat of her low-mileage 2011 Subaru Outback and not bound and gagged in the cargo hold. I was going to need that area for a few storage bins and some luggage.

I gave Mom the task of packing a couple of suitcases as if she were going on a trip. She needed her bathroom items, some clothes, and her unmentionables. In the meantime, I was packing other things up in storage bins. There were more clothes, her computer, her recent bills, and any tax records I could find.

I needed to grab some personal items from her apartment to incorporate into her new room in Texas. The thing about Mom was that she was good about hanging on to things that others would have jettisoned years ago.

Case in point was the collection of Tupperware tumblers in a variety of colors which brought back vivid memories of drinking non-adult beverages like milk and fruit punch.

Yeah those didn't come with us, but the picture cube did.

The picture cube was a pen/pencil holder which sat on Mom's desk for years, faithfully keeping just some of her pens and pencils in one centralized location. On each of the four exposed sides was a square picture from the old days: namely the 80s.

The first picture memorialized in true life and realistic color via Mom's Kodak is a picture featuring a plate of chocolate chip cookies strategically positioned in front of me, Thumper, and Chowsky. Chowsky, of course, was our big boy chow-malamute who had no problem striking a celebratory pose that says, "Look at what we used to feed the dog on his birthday back in the old days."

Back then, Chowsky would wash that down with a cool, refreshing drink of water from a porcelain bowl which was hooked up to its own water source in the bathroom.

For what it's worth, we never fed Chowsky or any of our other dogs chocolate. Rest assured that he was irritated to find out he had put forth the effort to pose in front of a plate of cookies he thought he would get to eat, only to find out he was given a piece of rawhide instead.

Rotate the cube a quarter turn (that's 90 degrees for the mathematically inclined) counter-clockwise and you're greeted with a picture of Ginger laying by the back door. Her German Shepherd markings blended well with the error-appropriate orange and brown carpeting that figured prominently throughout the house..

Turn the cube again to see a picture of Sunny. This yellow Labrador is only a puppy in the picture. The look on her face is one of guilt, as if she's just been caught on the bed when she wasn't supposed to be there.

And then, there's Chinook. The picture was taken on the same waterbed as the one of Sunny. Said bed is adorned with a white comforter with accent stripes in colors which remind you of that fast food burger franchise that used to suggest you could have it your way.

Chinook doesn't look guilty at all in that picture. That Malamute was born on third base and spent her whole life thinking she hit a triple. The thing about "Nookie" / "Wookie-noofers" was that she did have character. She had a habit of pushing all her kibble to the back of her bowl with her nose before she would eat it.

Rearranging her vittles was nothing compared to her other talent.

That dog talked.

A lot.

I mean, she didn't talk endlessly like a time traveling mad scientist trapped in the body of a nursing home resident or anything like that.

Instead, she had a habit of expressing herself with the phrase "Ahrooo-rooo-rooo", which loosely translated to "I hit a triple!"

Since that picture cube was a constant fixture in Mom's life, I made sure to include it with the personal items which were coming to Texas.

Sundown

There's a term for late day confusion in people with dementia called "sundowning".

Sundowning is an experience of increased confusion and agitation late in the day. It starts in late afternoon and can last well into the night. Anxiety and aggression can develop. Some people hallucinate, seeing or hearing things that aren't really there.

Weatherill RN CAEd, Gail . The Caregiver's Guide to Dementia: Practical Advice for Caring for Yourself and Your Loved One (Caregiver's Guides) (p. 53). Rockridge Press. Kindle Edition.

I didn't know that term back then, but I certainly witnessed it. Throughout the whole evening while I was trying to pack what needed to be packed, Mom was in a whole different world. It was like that call back in April that started all of this.

She couldn't stay on task and spent more time inspecting some of the different tops that she was packing. She spent time trying other tops on or changing her shoes. The little monster in my head was going nuts, and it was all I could do to put him away, bound and gagged in the cargo hold of a low-milage, 2011 Subaru Outback.

At one point, I took a break from my packing to go check on Mom. She had gone to bed.

I pulled out my phone and called up the group text I had with Wifey and Thumper. "If there was any doubt on whether we made the right call, rest assured that we did."

I loaded up the last storage bin into the car, went back upstairs, and laid down on the couch. The odor of Brandi's incontinence was ubiquitous.

Even still, I slept better that night than I had in months.

A Loaf Of Bread, A Jug Of Milk, A Gallon Of Gas

I woke up early that next morning. I had slept better that night than I had in months because I no longer had concerns about Mom being alone.

The smell of the unaddressed pet stains on the carpet permeated my senses.

After getting dressed, I started cleaning out her refrigerator. Save for the assorted sauces and condiments on the door and a couple of half gallons of mint chocolate chip ice cream in the freezer, it was empty.

As I finished, I felt a presence that I hadn't felt since....

I turned around and there was Mom standing there with a "what-in-tarnation are you doing" look on her face.

"Good morning," I greeted her.

"What are you doing?"

"I was just cleaning out the fridge here so that nothing goes bad. Are you ready to take a trip?" She just stared at me. "Okay, tell you what. I'm going to take this trash out and go gas up your car. Can you start getting ready to leave?"

"Yeah." Oh good. I wasn't going to have to tell her what we were doing again.

About a month ago, I had received a call from some highway courtesy service about Mom. She was stranded on the side of the road because her car wouldn't run. I spent the whole afternoon trying to contact Mom about the issue. I called her friend Cheryl as well. It seems that Mom had run out of gas, and Cheryl was trying to help her. Arguments had ensued and Cheryl was told to go away.

And Cheryl did exactly that.

On a Saturday morning a month later, I would gather more details around the gas issue.

The revelation came to me at pump five at the Loaf-n-Jug around the corner from apartment H.

Loaf-n-Jug.

What a name for an inconvenience store.

Once I figured out the gas cap was on the passenger side, the next riddle came with figuring out how to open its protective door.

There's nothing more frustrating than trying to read all the buttons, levers, and switches in an unfamiliar car which will keep you from carrying out a simple task. After minutes of button pushing, lever flipping, and switch flicking, I finally found the release lever on the floor in front of the driver's seat.

But wait.

There's more.

There was still an issue with getting gas into this low-mileage 2011 Subaru Outback.

Between finding which side the fill tube was on, and finding how to open the door, this was issue number three.

The lever wasn't working correctly and wouldn't open the gas door.

Let's summarize the last two days.

My flight out of San Antonio was delayed, and we had to swing out over Abilene to get to Dallas where I would be staying with my little brother, whose rental vehicle had been inappropriately towed because it had inappropriately been deemed to have been inappropriately parked when in fact it was appropriately parked.

Upon arriving in Colorado Springs, I was jettisoned from a Volkswagen Fahrvergnügen by a Somali pirate at the wrong apartment H. Even still I gave him a 5-star rating, because as a rule, you never want to down-vote a pirate.

Mom chose to sundown instead of packing last night.

Now, I can't get gas into her car.

If I can't get gas into this 2011 low-mileage Subaru Outback, we can't leave.

If we can't leave, I can't save Mom.

So what do I do?

Do I seek out a mechanic?

Do I pry it open and get it fixed once we get to Texas?

Better yet, do I rifle through that tool kit I saw in the back of the 2011 low-mileage Subaru Outback last night in hopes of finding some needle-nose goodness that will help me access the cable under that lever so that I can release the door?

Needless to say or should I say "needle-nose" to say, I was able to locate the appropriate tool to reach down in there under the fuel door release switch and pull the cable that would give me access to the fill tube.

I wonder if the pilot on that flight yesterday had to perform a similar maneuver so that more than enough jet fuel to get us out over Abilene could be added.

Irregardlessly, I wondered if the intrepid soul who invented needle-nose pliers ever encountered a similar situation which inspired their world-changing ingenuity.

When I got back to Mom's and announced that I went to the Loaf-n-Jug to gas up, she expressed her dislike for them. "They don't know how to open my gas cap."

<u>Irregardlessly</u>

There's something to be said about driving over 100 MPH (that's "miles per hour" for the uninitiated or those who pedantically demand precise language in discourse like this) on lightly traveled roads on the outskirts of town.

Don't do that.

It's dangerous.

It's stupid.

It's not behavior that 17-year-old boys should be engaging in, even though the story about three teachers being killed on this road a few years prior by a drunk driver still resonates.

Sometimes I would drive that fast in my own car on this road.

Sometimes I did it in Mom's medium-mileage, 1981 Oldsmobile Delta 88 with the diesel engine.

All these years later I hesitate to tell her I used to do that on Poison Spider Road. In the days when I was trafficking undeveloped film and printed pictures between the airport and several grocery stores, drug stores, and drive-thru photo booths like the one from the Twin Pines Mall where Doc Brown was assaulted by the Libyans for stealing their plutonium.

Those were the days when residents of the bustling metropolis of Casper, Wyoming had to send film off to Denver to be developed. Their anachronistic cell phones didn't feature a camera app yet.

All these years later, I was driving Mom's low-mileage, 2011 Subaru Outback with Mom firmly ensconced in the passenger seat wondering if I've gone a little mad for sweeping her away to Texas of all places.

Irregardlessly......

You may be wondering about that word and whether it constitutes good Englitch.

It probably doesn't.

"Irregardlessly" resides in the arsenal of words I use on the regular to see if anyone is paying attention to whatever it is I'm babbling about at any given point.

I do it so often that some of those voluntary verbal tics have become involuntary. For all tents and porpoises, I must stop myself and read the room sometimes just to make sure my audience is in an appropriate state of mind to recog-a-nize [sic] all my sic verbal behavior as intentional.

During the holidays when Mom tested positive for Covid and a trip for a two week, all-expense-paid relocation back into the hot zone wing at the nursing home where she originally started, I threw out the word "worserer", not thinking she was processing anything I was saying.

"Worserer?" she responded. It made my day when she questioned my grammar that way. It showed me that she understood that I was assaulting her native tongue in my own little way.

Back to that 11 or 12-hour drive to Texas, I threw out one of those words while avoiding conversation about how fast I used to drive her medium-mileage, 1981 Oldsmobile Delta 88 with the diesel engine on Poison Spider Road back in the old days.

Somewhere in the longitudinal middle of Colorado on the northbound side of I-25 (the opposite direction we were headed) we happened upon a vast field of solar panels, just lying around there in the sun, recharging their vitamin D levels.

"How about that?" I pontificated. "I always thought the components of those things were mined and assembled outside of the U.S. I didn't realize they were grown free-range here in the states.

Irregardlessly, I'm not sold on those things. Seems like they cost more money than they save you in the long run."

Mom just looked at me. "My dad used that word."

"Really? Prentiss Clyde Windsor, author of a master's thesis called <u>The Commoner in Shakespeare</u> and professor of Englitch literature at Angelo State University used the word 'irregardlessly'?"

"Englitch?" There was that look again.

"Did he use it with the same flair and irony that I do, or was that a verbal tick?"

"He did it on purpose."

"Well how 'bout that? I don't think I ever heard him say that."

I don't really have any additional stories from that part of the trip outside of the fact that we had some pretty good barbeque in Amarillo.

The only real purpose of this passage is to level set for some of the language in this odyssey which either has been or will be introduced.

Irregardlessly, you've been warned.

<u>Brenham Rhapsody</u>

Naturally, I wanted to get Mom moved out of Colorado Springs comfortably seated in the passenger seat and not bound and gagged in the cargo hold of her low-mileage, 2011 Subaru Outback. The best way I knew to do that was to include one specific item above all others on that trip.

Mom's luggage didn't matter and neither did mine.

Her current bills and other financial documents didn't matter.

Her laptop didn't matter.

All I needed in that car, besides Mom, was a debit card to cover the cost of gas, a pair of needle-nose pliers to pull that cable which would release the gas door, and the two half-gallons of Brenham's finest that had taken up the most space in Mom's empty freezer.

For the uninitiated, Blue Bell ice cream is produced in Brenham, Texas.

For purposes of this discussion, Brenham's finest in Mom's mind was Mint Chocolate Chip Ice Cream.

> *There's nothin like the taste of Blue Bell homemade ice cream,*
>
> *There's nothing like the taste of the very best*

It was Mom's favorite and had occupied about 90% of her food pyramid for the last several months.

If I was going to get any pushback from her on the twelve-hour journey out of Colorado, through Raton Pass and into New Mexico, across the hill-less country of the Texas Panhandle, and then onto Dallas, I needed a physical persuasion device in case my verbal skills faltered.

Thus the ice cream.

In some of the research I did leading up to that trip, I found that giving ice cream to dementia patients helps to remove some of the frustration they're experiencing with cognitive decline. I also found that their sense of taste tends to go, with a taste for sweets being one of the last to remain.

Sweet is a taste they still can enjoy. Ice cream is your friend.

Weatherill RN CAEd, Gail . The Caregiver's Guide to Dementia: Practical Advice
for Caring for Yourself and Your Loved One (Caregiver's Guides) (p. 67).
Rockridge Press. Kindle Edition.

Mom had loved ice cream for as long as I could remember. Whereas she may have been eating ice cream to alleviate the stress she was under, I tend to believe it was because she loved the stuff, and nothing else tasted good to her anymore.

Hey there's a Dairy Queen. We should stop.

Whatever that noise is, it needs to stop.

Why aren't we stopping for ice cream?

That noise is starting to bother me.

Here's a quick pop quiz.

How do you transport a couple of half gallon containers of Blue Bell Mint Chocolate Chip Ice Cream across state lines and keep it cold at the same time?

East bound and down, loaded up and truckin'

We gonna do what they say can't be done

Naturally, I couldn't seek out the services of Snowman, Fred the hound, Frog (complete with her wedding dress), and The Bandit.

After all, the drivers and the hound from that mission are no longer with us. Furthermore, the thought of towing a refrigerated trailer adorned with a beautiful mural of a stagecoach robbery behind Mom's low-mileage, 2011 Subaru Outback never crossed my mind.

Back when the boys were young, we didn't have a Dairy Queen in Casper until Randy was about 8 or 9. They were even a sponsor of the boys' Little League team.

There was one summer when it seems like I took the boys to Dairy Queen every afternoon. I couldn't get enough of that stuff, and neither could the boys.

What has Randy done to my car that it's making that awful squeaking noise?

Instead of using a refrigerated trailer, I purchased one of those Styrofoam coolers from a nearby grocery store and a couple bags of ice to house the ice cream for the next 12 hours.

Here's another quick pop quiz.

When you're transporting Blue Bell Mint Chocolate Chip Ice Cream in a low-mileage, 2011 Subaru Outback across state lines from Colorado, through New Mexico, and into Texas, and you're trying to keep it good and cold in one of those cheap Styrofoam coolers purchased in a local grocery store, how many times will you need to reach behind you into the cargo hold where the cooler is stored to adjust the lid so that it will stop making that infernal squeaking noise which is caused by the movements and vibrations of the car?

We eat all we can and we sell the rest,

It's all made, homemade down home

Let me assure you the stereo in a low-mileage, 2011 Subaru Outback does not get loud enough to drown that noise out.

Randy would always get a chocolate sundae, and more times than not he would dribble chocolate sauce on his shirt because he was talking while eating.

Okay, he's fixed the noise. Good. That was starting to bother me.

Ever since Blue Bell showed up in Colorado about 10 years ago, I haven't been able to get enough of it.

Now, it's all I eat.

Oh, there's that noise again.

<u>Dallas At Midnight</u>

The day had started off what felt like about 48 hours ago when I woke up on Mom's couch with the odoriferous remains of Brandi's incontinence executing a devastating assault on my olfactory nerve.

There was that issue with the gas cap, and then the late start, and then breakfast at my least favorite fast-food joint in the whole wide world that kept us from getting on the road before 11a.m.

Twelve hours later we had traversed Colorado, the northeastern corner of New Mexico, and the endless horizons in the flat Panhandle of Texas. We were now making our way east to Dallas.

It's late and we've been on the road all day.

Randy wouldn't even let me drive.

This morning, I woke up to noises in my apartment. I've had a lot of visitors coming in and going out at all hours of the day lately. I just assumed it was one of them.

When I got up to go confront them and tell them to quiet down, I found Randy throwing away everything in the fridge. He better not have touched my ice cream, or I'll take the orange paddle to him.

He gave me some story about not wanting my food to spoil while we're gone.

Gone?

Gone from where?

Where could we be going so that my food is going to spoil?

Randy mentions something about needing to put gas in my car. Fine with me, that means I don't have to pay for it. I hope he doesn't go to that place around the corner where they don't know how to open my gas door. They made me run out of gas once out on the highway.

That was this morning.

The plan was to spend the night in Dallas with Thumper, my little brother and Mom's other favorite son. We were then going to eat brunch with him and his friends the next morning, go introduce Mom to her new great grandson, and then head home to San Antonio.

Finding the right exit to get to Thumper's downtown apartment at midnight, in an unfamiliar city, using a navigation option on my phone which was baffled by the confuse-opoly of a freeway system was kind of like looking for a gas door release switch on a low-mileage, 2011 Subaru Outback so that you can evacuate a loved one who is in cognitive decline.

I overshot my turn three or four times that night while Thumper was texting me asking where I was.

"Your first mistake was staking up ground in this hellhole," I told him at one point when he called, dispensing with any sort of greeting. "You hate their football team as much as I do. Why would you want to live in the land of the enemy? I'll call you back in a few minutes when I make the right turn." I then hung up without giving him a chance to talk.

Now, I'm not even sure I know where we are. I just know it's not Colorado. Randy is getting upset because he can't find his way around town. He keeps arguing with someone on the phone and repeating about how much he hates Dallas.

Are we in Dallas?

I have family there.

America's team, my ass.

Ten minutes later, we were in the vicinity of his apartment, and I called him back. Pleasantries were exchanged and we proceeded to gameplan our next step.

Thumper was outside hoping to spot and flag me down. After twelve hours of driving, I was hoping to spot him before I ran him down.

Finally, our longitude and latitude converged, and he pointed me into the parking garage for his apartment complex. Just two days prior, the management of said complex inappropriately deemed Thumper's rental vehicle to have been inappropriately parked in said garage and had it towed and impounded.

Randy was arguing with someone on the phone while driving. Why was he so mad? Whoever it is, he just hung up on him. "There he is..."

My concern was whether the management would inappropriately deem a certain low-mileage, 2011 Subaru Outback to be inappropriately parked so they could also have it towed and impounded.

As we pulled into the garage and ascended to the second floor, Thumper ran out ahead of us to guide us to our ultimate destination.

Understand the following immutable facts.

Thumper and I are built the same way.

Fire plugs with no necks shouldn't run.

Who waves at a car in the middle of the night? "Run fat boy run!" *What did you just say?*

Yeah, I shouldn't have said that. I told Mom as much when she stared at me for committing such a verbal indiscretion in a volume loud enough to hear.

Why is he chasing that person?

Whoever he's following is now guiding us into a parking spot. "We're here."

Where's 'here'?

Whoever Randy was just chasing has opened my door and is now coming after me.

Who is that?

As we parked, we found that Thumper's best friend and her boyfriend were there to greet and assist. After twelve hours on the road, I could use the relief. The saving grace was that Mom has a relationship with Thumper's best friend, so it's not like some strange lady was fawning all over her.

Oh, that's Bobby.

I was thinking about moving in with Bobby some time ago. Is that what I'm doing now?

"Take these two bags and grab that infernal Styrofoam cooler. I have her ice cream in there and it needs time in the freezer."

Ice cream?

Bobby's friends are holding onto me for dear life.

Why are they doing that?

Oh look, there's Brandi. Why is she barking at Randy?

No, wait. That's not Brandi. What's that dog's name?

After getting Mom into the apartment and all squared away, we made plans for the next day and called it a night.

That reminds me. I need to go pick up Brandi's ashes tomorrow. I tried to pick them up yesterday, but they wouldn't give them to me.

I'll get them tomorrow. I'm going to bed.

The Next Four Weeks

<u>Coins & Cards</u>

Twenty-four hours later, Mom and I arrived at my house in her low-mileage, 2011 Subaru Outback.

Last night we were in downtown Dallas, and I was yelling at Thumper on the phone while warding off quizzical and sometimes accusatory glares from the owner of the vehicle who was seated comfortably in the passenger seat and not bound and gagged in the cargo hold. There was a chance that the attitude I displayed back then would have been introduced as evidence of the vehicular fratricide I considered committing that night.

Spoiler alert.

Thumper survived and bought us brunch the next day.

Afterward, we drove out to one of the 'burbs to meet up with Mom's freshly minted great-grandson. After a few short naps on Mom's part, we headed south for San Antonio.

I would like to say the mere fact that I showed up on Mom's doorstep in Colorado one day and said, "Let's go", followed up by successfully getting her to Texas and under my roof constituted a "Mission Accomplished" banner.

"Mission Accomplished", in the sense that phase one was complete, and several unforeseen and unplanned phases were about to ensue.

Looking back, the first phase of getting Mom to Texas in her low-mileage, 2011 Subaru Outback was the easiest part of the mission.

I had to figure out how to take over the management of her life since she wasn't doing that anymore.

I had to figure out how to get her the medical care she needed.

I had to expand her diet beyond the primary export of the cattle in Brenham, Texas where Mom's favorite ice cream is produced.

I had to figure out how to get her moved out of apartment H in Colorado Springs.

I had to figure out what to do with her.

Over that first week, I gained access to her laptop and phone and systematically reconstructed her finances. Wifey started working on Mom's diet. Our two dogs, Faith and Charlie, offered up their own kind of support as well.

I really, really wish that were all we had to do.

One night I was in the back room reading with Charlie the Silver Labrador at my side. She was helping me sound out the big words.

Wifey appeared out of nowhere with a panicked look on her face. "Your Mom is going through our purses!"

"Really? You don't have anything to hide, do you?" That triggered a non-Mom glare from my beloved wife of nearly thirty years which even caused Charlie to flinch.

"Can you come get her?"

Wifey and Juniorette were in the habit of keeping their purses on the table by the door. When I got there, Mom was going through them. "Hey Mom, whatcha doin'?"

"I'm looking for Iditarod Coins."

"Iditarod Coins? What are those?"

"I don't know."

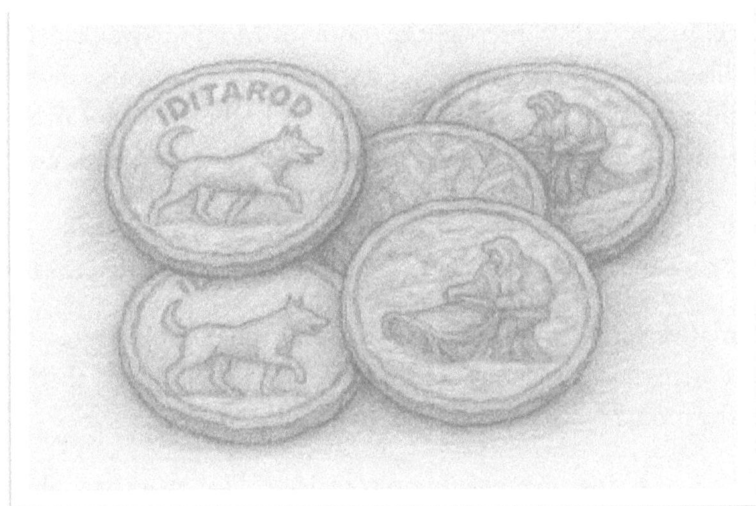

"Okay, well do you think they may be in your purse in your room? Neither of these purses are yours."

"Okay." I took Mom to her room to find her purse. Out of the corner of my eye, I could see Wifey's and Juniorette's purses being swiftly evacuated by their respective owners.

As I walked away with Mom, I brought up a potentially touchy subject. "You know Mom, I need to fly back to Colorado and work on getting your apartment packed up. Do you have any thoughts about what you want to do with your furniture?"

"I don't want you going through my things like that," said the woman who had spent the last several minutes rifling through purses which weren't hers.

A few days later I found Mom sitting at the old desk we had in the room prior to her arrival.

I had scattered several pictures and old concert tickets on the top of the desk under its protective glass.

All things being equal, I'm fairly sure the desk belonged to Grandma.

Irregardlessly, I had a few odds and ends in there which were not of any major importance. In the rush to prepare the room for Mom's arrival, we didn't really bother to liberate it from my old charging cables, watch bands, novelty playing cards, flashlights, old wallets, checkbooks, thumbtacks, envelopes, postage stamps, or an 18-year-old cigar gifted to me when one of my nephews arrived.

Mom's search for the Iditarod Coins expanded to the drawers in that desk. I had an old checkbook register stashed in there that she decided to review.

In my formative years, Mom was militant about me keeping a register for my accounts. Furthermore, she insisted that I keep it balanced and that I reconcile it against the monthly statements from the bank.

Seeing her inspecting my checkbook register like that brought back an unpleasant memory or two. At the same time, I became hopeful that she could find that $0.17 out-of-balance issue I was tracking down a few days before.

It was doubtful she would find anything in that checkbook, because here in the 21st century, I don't track my finances manually using medieval witchcraft such as handwriting, a check register, or arithmetic.

"How's it going Mom?"

"Oh fine." Mom put down the register and picked up a deck of playing cards which featured pictures of dogs taken with a fish-eye lens. "I bought these cards a few years ago at a gift shop in The Springs."

For the uninitiated, people from Colorado Springs and the vicinity refer to their hometown as "The Springs". I've never heard any of my neighbors in San Antonio use the same sort of abbreviation, so maybe I should get something started on that.

"The dogs on them are so cute, I just couldn't resist. I've had this deck for a while and am looking forward to playing games with them."

"Sounds like a plan. It would seem to me there's only one game you should play with a deck of cards like that, where some of those dogs are bound to be fixed females."

"Spades?" Okay, I didn't expect Mom to know the punchline to my spontaneous Dad joke.

"Spades."

The deck of cards in question was one of three decks I had stashed in that desk. I bought it years ago when Wifey, the kids and I were playing a lot of poker.

I bought it at a grocery store here in The Antonio.

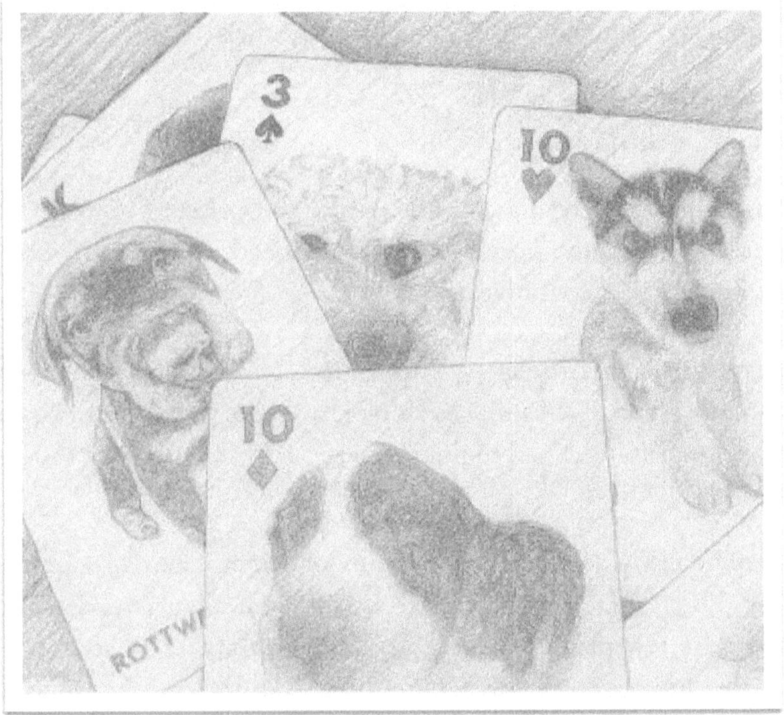

There Where The Ware Was

There's something to be said for moving someone out of their home when they're unable to participate in the process.

On top of all the challenges of getting Mom moved in with me, we also had to get her moved out of apartment H in Colorado Springs.

A few weeks ago, right around lunch time on a Friday, Mom and I had given notice at the Enchanted Springs Apartment Complex that she would be relinquishing her command by the end of September.

In the next ten weeks, we had to get everything out of the apartment. Furthermore, we had to manage the move-out from one thousand miles away.

Going further, we were trying to move to the next phase of Mom's life where we had to get her to resume a normal diet. We then had to gameplan how we were going to deal with her cognitive decline.

Taking care of the apartment was 4th or 5th on my list of priorities where Mom was concerned. Even still, I couldn't just ignore it in favor of having more important things to do. I had to figure out what to do with everything she had in there.

She had standard-issue furniture in the living room. She had a propane grill and some patio furniture out on the balcony. She had two desks, two file cabinets, and a few printers in one of the bedrooms. She had a table and a hutch in the dining room. She had a washer and dryer in the laundry closet. She had a dresser, a chest of drawers, and a waterbed complete with several gallons of water and three-piece headboard set in the bedroom. She had several bookshelves adorned with books and other knickknackery which was present in my youth. She had clothes in the closets of both bedrooms. She had hardware in the closet and a kitchen which was fully stocked with all the cookware, bakeware, drinkware, flatware, silverware, and Tupperware that one could ever use.

Steven Wright said it best. "You can't have everything. Where would you put it?"

I would need to take a minimum of three more trips to Colorado Springs to get Mom moved out of apartment H.

On the first trip I would get everything ready to move out. I would identify what had to come back, what might be able to come back, and what couldn't come back to Texas.

On the second trip, I would conscript a brute squad from within the family tree to fly up there with me, rent a moving truck, and drive back with the items which were coming back.

On the third trip, I would sell, donate, or trash (not necessarily in that order) whatever was left.

Fortunately, Mom was there to help.

Kind of.

Three years ago, after doing her estate planning, Mom had penned (okay, typed up) a document outlining all the keepsakes in her apartment which I should watch out for in case she croaks.

Her words, not mine.

The document was titled "THINGS TO KNOW IN CASE I CROAK".

I had nearly forgotten about this breadcrumb until I found it on her laptop while I was reconstructing her finances and trying to figure out how to take care of her.

My lowest points in the entire ordeal of getting Mom the care she needed came from those subsequent trips to apartment H.

I didn't want to go rifle through all of Mom's things and make decisions about everything that was in that apartment, but it had to be done.

I had to go through her files to grab what I needed, shred the sensitive stuff I didn't need, and toss the rest.

I had to go through her books to grab what I wanted and donate the rest.

I had to go through her kitchen making decisions on cookware, bakeware, drinkware, flatware, silverware, and Tupperware to keep, and what to let go.

I had to go through her wall hangings and match them up to the "THINGS TO KNOW IN CASE I CROAK" document to determine if they had sentimental or other value.

I had to go through all the knickknackery and make decisions about what to keep and what to let go.

I had to go through the closets in both bedrooms and make decisions on what clothes she could use in Texas.

Between each one of those decisions on that first trip, I was fielding communiques from Wifey about how Mom wasn't doing so good.

All throughout, the odoriferous remnants of Brandi's incontinence permeated the apartment.

Every single piece of it was overwhelming.

And then, part one was done, and I could go back home.

Naturally, my return flight wasn't free of any additional nuance or nuisance. In this case, it was accented with a publicly broadcasted message which was meant specifically for me.

The message didn't come by way of a flight delay which would force us to swing out over Abilene to avoid some weather.

There were no unforeseen circumstances that would force me to stay the night in Dallas again.

There was no need to go chase down a rental vehicle that had been inappropriately deemed to have been inappropriately parked and subsequently and inappropriately impounded.

There were no more repeated attempts to find the right exit to get to Thumper's downtown apartment at midnight either.

Instead, the subtle, non-verbal message I got while waiting for a connecting flight from Dallas to San Antonio came from a fellow sojourner.

Put very simply, the message came from a lady wearing a lot of headware.

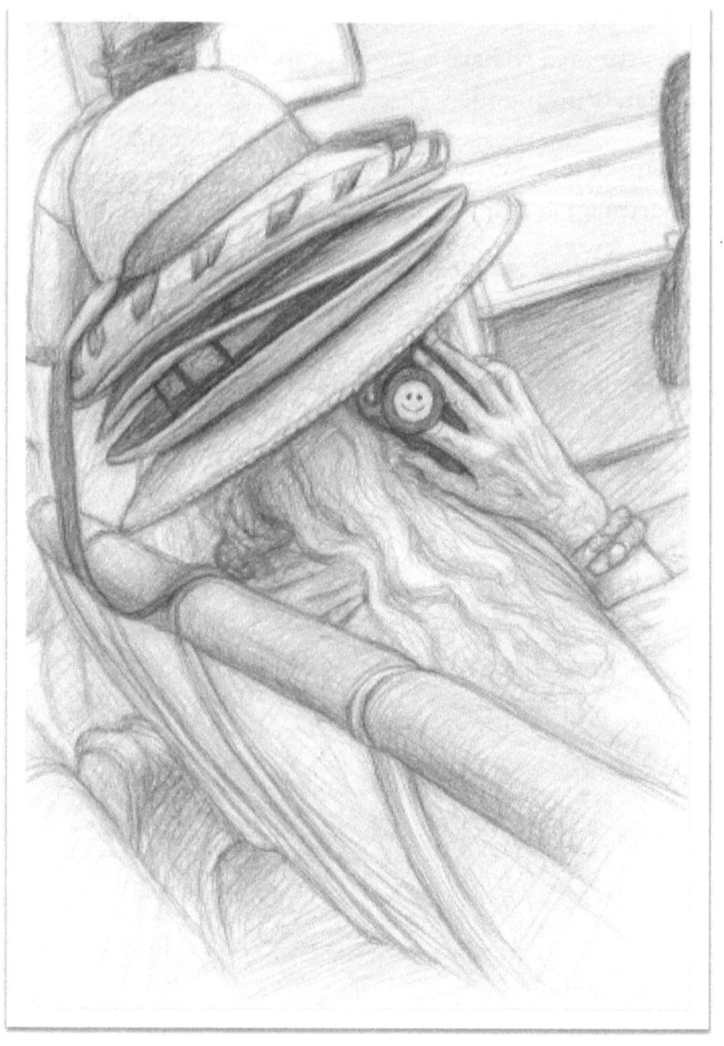

To the untrained eye, the message was nothing but the absurdity of someone waiting for the same flight back home, utilizing the most efficient method available to transport either four single layer hats or one hat with four layers, all at the same time atop a tuft of golden tresses.

For me, the message was something else.

When it came to taking care of Mom, I was putting on too many hats.

I was trying to be her business manager, her caretaker, her dietician, and her son all at the same time.

Things were about to get worserer.

<u>The BSOD</u>

There comes a point in all our lives when we add so many programs, processes, functionalities, and features to our computers that things become problematic.

Next to the virus and anti-virus software, there's also cleanup utilities, assorted cloud backups, instant messaging, weather updates, and other collections of code designed to make your life easier and harder all at the same time.

It's just enough bells and whistles to make some unwanted noise.

If the computer is not designed to handle all the noise, the device bogs down.

The performance falters and the processing speed becomes glacial.

The next thing you know, the computer gives you the Blue Screen Of Death (BSOD) which admonishes you that it's had enough.

Leaving Mom at home with Wifey during that long weekend so I could go pack up apartment H created two BSOD's.

One of those BSOD's happened with Wifey who had been overwhelmed with handling Mom.

The other BSOD was Mom.

If I could look back for that moment in time when Mom's decline went into overdrive, it was that last weekend in July when I left for a few days.

It was late Monday night at the end of July, and my plane had just touched down in San Antonio.

Wifey and I had texted back and forth over the last several days, so I was under no illusion that everything would be fine when I got home.

Mom had stayed in bed all weekend. She didn't leave that bed for any reason, whatsoever.

Once I got home, Wifey and I tried to convince her to get out of bed so that we could take care of the most basic of her needs.

"DON'T TOUCH ME OR I WILL KICK YOU!"

"Please do. That will give me assurance that you can still move."

I was tired. I had just spent the last four days in apartment H making decisions I didn't want to make. I had just gotten off the plane where I had been in the air all day. It was late and I was in no mood. To this day I don't know how I managed to remain calm when Mom yelled at me like that.

Where have you been and why are you talking to me that way?

Of course I can move!

Wait.

I can't move.

Okay this isn't dementia or senility or anything like that. Those are mental issues; this is a physical one.

I've got entities again. I can tell without even muscle testing.

You probably didn't smudge the house or even this room to let the positive energies in did you?

Look, I know you don't believe in this stuff, but I do, okay? I assure you it was an entity that made me fall down the stairs at my apartment a few years ago. It was an entity that got to me when you and I were out walking your dog once too.

It's an entity this time, and I'm going to take care of it.

> *Oh Divine Spirit, I implore you to close portals to all evil, darkness, and negativity, and from time, space, dimensions, and realities. Only allow energy that is the light or from the light, to pass through.*

I believe in the eternal Goodness, the eternal Loving-kindness, and the eternal Givingness of Life to all.

And so it is!

Okay I think it's gone now. I should be better tomorrow morning.

We got her out of bed and cleaned up.

Managing Mom's physical needs over the next two weeks boiled down to moving her back and forth between the bed, an office chair (eventually replaced with a wheelchair), the bathroom, and the recliner.

Mom never walked on her own again.

Convalescence

By mid-August, I managed to get a home nursing service to visit and make an assessment. Wifey and I weren't equipped or trained to provide the type of physical care Mom needed, and we weren't doing her or ourselves any favors.

The results of that assessment, as troubling as they were, came as a welcome relief.

"I don't mean to be rude here," said the cocky young doctor with the shaggy hair. "...but you two are way out of your element here."

Oh thank God. My internal monologue had turned the volume knobs up to eleven.

"She's dehydrated and malnourished. We'll need to admit her so we can get her stabilized."

Stabilized? I'm fine.

Earlier that day, one of the visiting nurses strongly suggested we get her to an emergency room. A little while later, as I was preparing to lift Mom into the passenger seat of her low-mileage, 2011 Subaru Outback, she made one of the last coherent statements she would ever make. "I don't want to go."

"I'm sorry Mom, I know you don't want to go. I know that visiting an emergency room or a hospital is the last thing you want to do. I know that you abhor western medicine. I also know that you're in bad shape right now. Do you remember the doctor who came to the house to see you last week? She said you have a UTI. Since then we haven't been able to get you to take medication for it."

But I did muscle testing on that and cleared it. I don't have a UTI now.

"We can't get you to eat."

I'm not hungry.

"We can barely get you to drink."

I'm not thirsty.

"We're tired, and we don't know how to take care of you anymore. We need to get you to someone who can. I promise you that I will not allow any invasive treatments beyond getting you better."

You promised me you wouldn't do this to me when I made you my power of attorney and executor. Don't forget your promise!

—I won't Mom.

Mom looked at me for a moment with the same gaze she gave me when I asked her to move to Texas.

"Okay."

Los Prados Verdes Center for Nursing & Rehabilitation

<u>Room 209</u>

September 1st couldn't get here any faster.

Mom had been admitted to the hospital in mid-August. Once she was stabilized, it became clear she'd need to move to a nursing facility for recovery care. The snag: her Medicare plan only covered providers in Colorado, not Texas.

The hospital and nursing facility tried to arrange a short-term contract so her care would be covered until her new Texas-based plan began on September 1st. That contract never came through—lost somewhere between dropped balls and red tape—so Mom spent the rest of August in the hospital before transferring to Los Prados Verdes Center for Nursing & Rehabilitation once the new coverage took effect.

Just on background, "Los Prados Verdes" translates to "I changed the name of the nursing facility to protect the privacy of the cast of characters Mom and I interacted with because I didn't change many of their names in the process."

When I got Mom to Texas and spent a few weeks wondering what I was going to do with her, I never had the intention of getting her in a nursing home. After all, we thought she didn't need such care. We never saw the possibility that her arrival in Texas would usher in her mental and physical shutdown.

Yet now, here she was lying in a bed in the wing reserved for new and quarantined residents.

Thank you Covid.

Mom's arrival at Prados Verdes came at the tail-end of the lockdown and its associated mask [sic] hysteria. She couldn't move her legs and was barely moving her arms. She couldn't feed herself or do anything else for that matter.

After being cleared from the quarantine after 10 days, Mom was moved to another wing for a short time before she was eventually moved to a more permanent residence in room 209.

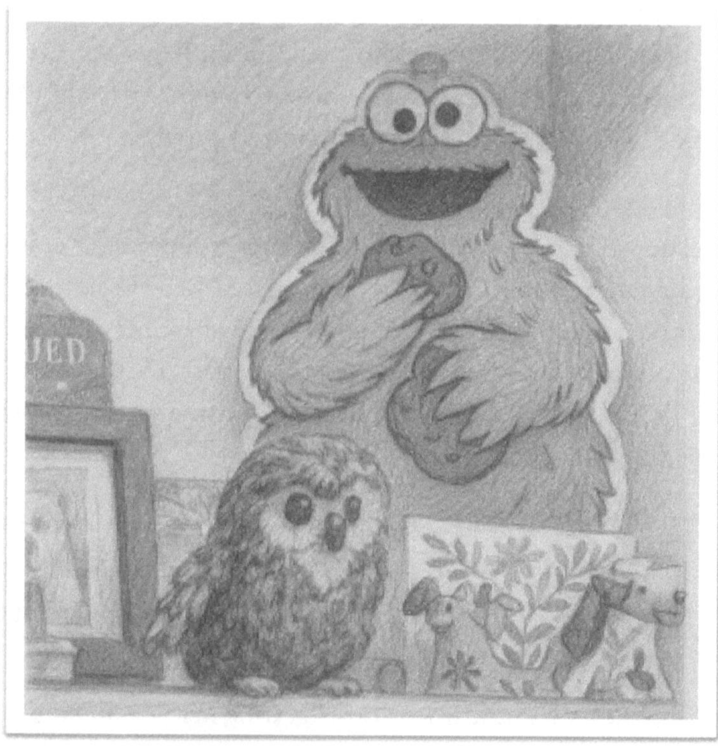

We filled the room with assorted pictures of her dogs, her kids, her grandkids, her great grandkid, a Cookie Monster pennant we got at some ice show we attended at McNichols arena in Denver back in the 70's, and some other knickknackery. The famed and framed picture of Barb out back the Outback in her Outback took up a position which hinted to staff that even though their charge in room 209 didn't say or do a whole lot, she had a sense of humor.

<u>The Nurses Station</u>

With Mom's situation now stabilized at Los Prados Verdes Center for Nursing & Rehabilitation, I developed a new set of rituals.

Given that Mom was living just a matter of minutes away from my office, I started visiting her after work. I would make sure the TV in her room was broadcasting some food-oriented program in hopes that she would get inspired to eat whatever pureed nourishment that landed in front of her on any given day.

One day in October, after Mom had been at Prados Verdes for about a month, I arrived to find that she wasn't in her room.

Well crud.

She can't leave on her own. What have these people done with my Mom?

Had something happened?

Why didn't they call me?

What have these people done with my Mom?

I walked down the hall to the nurses station to find out what was going on.

Contrary to my initial expectation, the nurses station wasn't manned (or wo-manned, take your pick) by a gaggle of scrub-clad individuals charged with the well-being of the residents here at Prados Verdes.

The bulk of the staff which was clad in scrubs were Certified Nursing Assistants (C.N.A.'s), and they had been dispatched to rooms up and down the hall to get the residents ready for dinner. One Registered Nurse (RN) was behind the circular desk doing whatever it is that RNs do in places like these.

Surrounding the desk was a majestic herd of residents in varying states of dress from stretchy two-piece jammies to house coats, to business professional attire. There were about ten of them, stationed around that desk and they were just staring at the RN.

They were not talking.

Correction.

One of them was talking.

A lot.

I was a little gobsmacked that she didn't have an oxygen supply, as the speed and longevity at which she jabbered allowed for no pause to take in a breath or two.

The shock of white hair and her rapid-fire speech—easily pushing eighty-eight miles per hour—reminded me of a movie character. In my mind, she was Doc Brown.

Walking up on this scene was a bit confusing.

Oh good you're here. I was beginning to think you'd never show up. This lady will not shut up.

Was Doc Brown breathlessly sharing her vast knowledge and experiences with her colleagues, neighbors, friends, and all others who had gathered around for additional inspiration?

Better yet, was Doc Brown dispensing coded messages via her recursive rambling to her fellow co-conspirators?

Let's get out of here before someone notices this horrendous dress they've put on me.

I stood there for a few moments taking in the view while attempting to translate what Doc Brown was saying.

Over the years I'd developed a specific set of skills for processing two kinds of difficult audio.

First: English spoken with a heavy accent by someone who clearly wasn't using their primary language. I'd been on plenty of conference calls where the geographical location of the participants wasn't limited to the lower forty-eight.

Second: audio delivered at double speed. I picked that up early in my career, when I had to review tape-recorded telemarketer calls to make sure the fine print was covered. With the sheer volume of calls, listening at twice the speed was the only way to keep up with my workload.

Randy?

Even though I still use that skill today to get through all the daily podcasts I subscribe to, I found my talent to be lacking when it came to interpreting the high-speed data stream Doc Brown was transmitting.

Hey Randy, I'm over here.

Certainly, I could pick out a lot of what she was saying and mentally fill in the rest to get the context of it all. That's what I do when someone talks to me in Spanish.

Even still, I was having a difficult time picking out any one idea that Doc Brown was sharing.

RANDY!

As I stood there succumbing to the siren sounds of Doc Brown, I experienced a twinge I hadn't felt since...

There was a time in my formative years in which half-ass attempts at performing my chores were met with disdain, derision, and other alliteration. When this happened, Mom would appear out of nowhere to compel my conversion of half-assed work to full-assed work.

She would stand there with her arms folded, jettison her need or ability to blink, and just glare at Thumper or me until the leaves were raked, the carpet was vacuumed, the wood was stacked, or the snow in the driveway was shoveled.

Sitting right there at the 11 o'clock position from the RN's point of view was Mom. She was slathered in that terrifying dress that I had yet to carelessly, yet purposely, transition to the on-site incinerator. I could only guess how long she had been there, wearing that dress— that spate of troublesome technicolor—while being subjected to Doc Brown's monotonous monologues.

Like all the residents seated around that station, Mom was glaring at the RN with that same look of derision over half-assed versus full-assed work. This led me to believe that Mom and the others had not voluntarily gathered around with bated breath and great anticipation to take in all that Doc Brown had to share.

Much like being trapped on a crowded elevator after someone has passed gas, Mom and her colleagues, neighbors, and friends had been involuntarily deposited there for guerrilla story time.

More importantly, Mom was out of bed and in a wheelchair. This was a pleasant surprise, as I could now take her outside for a walk occasionally.

"Excuse me," I called out to the RN.

"Yes?"

"This is the first time I know of where Mom's been out of bed or out of her room. Can you tell me what's going on?"

"Oh we've started taking her to the dining room with some of the other residents who need help with their eating. Once we get them out of bed and ready to eat, we just bring them here until it's time to go to the dining room."

"Ah, that makes sense. The way they're all just staring at you, I thought they were supervising your work."

<u>Avoiding My Mistakes</u>

From: Randy Tharp

Sent: Sunday, September 25, 2022, 9:04 A.M.

To: Dar-Dar (*my son attached this name to one of his aunts when he was learning to talk*),

Laka-Laka (*my son ascribed this name to his aunt which could talk as fast as Doc Brown*)

Subject: Long Term Care

Howdy.

While I was at your mom's yesterday conducting acts of technical wizardry (hitting CTRL+ALT+DELETE) and further instilling in your collective minds the silly notion that I'm an "IT Guy", the discussion of preventative measures came up.

In the process of taking over the management of my mom's life in the last three months, I've picked up a few tidbits which will serve you well if/when your Mom should become incapacitated. I understand you already have some of these items in place, however I'm going to list them anyway just to make sure they've been said aloud.

My hope here is that by sharing some of the experiences I've had recently, you'll avoid them in the future. Translation: Learn from my mistakes.

Estate Planning:

- Know where she keeps these items and maintain copies of your own.

- Will
- Power of Attorney
- Medical Power of Attorney
- Advance directive

- HIPAA Authorization

Management of daily life:

- Make sure one of you has access to her bank account(s) and can sign on it.
- Know where all her passwords are, especially if she pays her bills online.
    - I was shown a little notepad yesterday with them all written down. Rest assured that will give you (and your purported "IT Guy") headaches. Navigating handwritten notes in a notepad for sites she may/may not be active on will not be fun.
    - Consider getting her a password application that retains that stuff. If you don't go this route, at least list the passwords on a Word/Excel document that's password protected. Just know what the password is to open that document, and where that document is located.

Long term care insurance:

- Medicare will not cover a nursing home stay.
- Medicaid will cover it.
    - You'll have to demonstrate that she has no resources to pay for care.
    - If she does have resources, don't try to hide them. That's fraud.
    - If you should pursue Medicaid, hire an advocate who will stay on top of the application process for you. There are too many moving parts involved to do that alone.
- Pursue long term care insurance.
    - This type of insurance is designed to pay for nursing care (home or facility)
    - It's recommended that you look into a policy around age sixty.

- I sought out a policy for my mom early this year when I started seeing memory issues (she's 78)
    - She was denied for the first policy we tried because the person who evaluated her could see the immediate future. At least that's my guess. That was about $450 a month, and I'm guessing part of the cost was due to her age. It would have been cheaper if we had done this earlier.
    - We were able to get her approved for a supplemental policy at around $350 a month. It doesn't have all the bells and whistles, but it should take care of her immediate needs.
    - I know this sounds expensive as a monthly rate, however the daily rate for Mom's room is $255 a day which is around $7K a month. Mom's policy allows for $300 a day, so that monthly premium is worth it.

I think I've covered the main items here, but if you have further questions, let me know.

Best and warmest regards,

The Purported IT Guy

Officially signed with the initials of one of the great grandsons of an outstandingly Prominent Citizen.

RGT

From: Dar-Dar

Sent: Sunday, September 30, 2022, 12:48 P.M.

To: Randy Tharp

Subject: Long Term Care

Thanks for the info Randy!

Dar-Dar

From: Laka-Laka

Sent: Sunday, September 30, 2022, 12:52 P.M.

To: Randy Tharp

Subject: Long Term Care

Randy you dropped into my spam folder...

Thank you.

From: Randy Tharp

Sent: Sunday, September 30, 2022, 1:30 P.M.

To: Laka-Laka

Subject: Long Term Care

Right where I was aiming.....

Officially signed with the initials of one of the great grandsons of an outstandingly Prominent Citizen.

RGT

First In First Out

Ellen was one of the many residents in the dining room.

She wore purple cat-eyeglasses, complete with a beaded garrote attached to the earpieces and gracefully draped around the back of her neck.

She talked with a slur which led me to believe that she had a stroke recently.

She was always decked out nicely in a dress.

She had a fastidious way about her where she would constantly adjust her dress to avoid showing too much leg.

Ellen was a sweetheart.

Ellen had control of her arms and legs; however she was always in a wheelchair. I really had to wonder whether her frail body could even bear the weight of her 80-pound frame, so perhaps it was better she didn't try walking.

Ellen was always a ray of sunshine unless her blood sugar was low. In those times, she became a little combative, but not so much that you felt that she was going to bop you upside the head or chew you out.

The thing about Ellen in that dining room is that she was usually the first one to get out of there once dinner started. She would barely eat her dinner and then scamper out of there. After all, she was in a rush to get her nighttime meds on board in time to watch an episode of *Matlock* and then call it a day.

On a few occasions, she got out of there before dinner arrived, thinking she had already eaten.

One evening, after getting Mom back to her room from the dining room where she had dined on pureed lasagna and a bowl of chocolaty goodness, I said good night and exited room 209. Halfway down the hall I encountered Ellen, seated in her chair, hanging on for dear life to the rails mounted to the walls. She was using her legs to propel her forward.

"Hi Ellen."

She looked up at me, twisted her head a little, adjusted her jaw side to side and squinted. "Will you push me?"

"Sure, where are we going?"

"To my room."

Yeah I didn't know where her room was, and she wasn't very sure either.

One time while I was in room 209 with Mom, Ellen tried to wheel her way in thinking she was at home. One of the C.N.A.'s just happened to be walking by at the time, so she stopped to pull Ellen's chair (with her in it), out of there. "Sorry about that." she said.

"Oh there's no harm. Ellen was just about to tell us a joke." I replied.

Randy, that's not funny.

—Sure it is. Let's see if she plays along.

The C.N.A. looked at her. "Ellen, were you going to tell Miss Barb a joke?"

Ellen didn't seem to suffer fools and put on an air of exasperation. "No."

Over the following months I would greet Ellen on a regular basis either in the dining room or in the hallway. At one point, she began calling me "Sweetheart".

"Look at that Mom, Ellen just called me 'Sweetheart.'"

Mom smirked. *Yeah, I noticed. She must not know you very well.*

The President of the Residents

When Mom was assigned to her permanent duty station in room 209 at Los Prados Verdes Center for Nursing & Rehabilitation, she found herself across the hall from room 208.

I know that sounds a bit coincidental, but that's how room numbers work in most buildings nowadays.

The resident of room 208 was none other than Linda.

Linda was the only resident on the north side of the building that made use of her bipedal mobility with the assistance of a walker she didn't really need. There was also a tank of nitrous attached to the superfluous walker which fed a tube directly to her nose. This gave Linda that extra edge if she needed to act on a moment's notice.

Okay, it was probably oxygen.

Linda was one of the only residents on the north side of the building that had avoided cognitive decline.

Linda had assigned duties which went beyond staring at the TV all day. Unlike the other residents, she didn't have to sit still for daily care.

She delivered mail to the residents who were still in the practice of receiving physical correspondence. She also ran the nightly bingo game where she called out numbers and executed swift justice on the more strident residents who resorted to fisticuffs over whether 'L32' was a real square.

She was also in charge of getting decorations hung up to celebrate all the major and minor holidays. That included decorating the doors of residents who couldn't decorate themselves.

Linda was the resident whose network could provide the other residents with cigarettes, a bag of reefer if that was their thing, a bottle of brandy to celebrate their grandkids' high school graduation, or anything else that was within reason.

Linda was the only guilty resident at Prados Verdes.

Linda also ran the betting pool among staff on how many residents would matriculate on any given day. Her real profit from that pool came from the bets on who would go and on what day.

Upon arriving one afternoon to help Mom with dinner, I happened upon Linda sitting in the lobby next to where I needed to sign in. "Hi Linda. Did someone send you to the office to talk to the principal?"

She didn't even acknowledge my little joke. "No, there's an advisory board meeting in a few minutes and I represent the residents."

This didn't really come as a surprise given her tenure and the tendrils she had on the daily operations of Los Prados Verdes Center for Nursing & Rehabilitation.

I placed a small wager with her, wished her luck in the upcoming meeting, and headed for room 209 to see Mom.

Later, Mom and I were sitting in our assigned seats in the dining room. The speakers overhead continued to pipe in music from my formative years.

The scent of barbeque was ubiquitous as the kitchen commandos prepared the properly pureed and plopped portions for each tray. Once all the residents were in place and the nursing staff could give the kitchen a headcount, dinner would be served.

Can I sail through the changing ocean tides?

Can I handle the seasons of my life?

As most of the other residents were being wheeled in by staff, Linda and her top lieutenant Gwendolyn arrived on their own accord. Linda was pushing her nitrous infused walker, and Gwendolyn was in her highly equipped motorized wheelchair which came standard with zero turn radius and an optional mulching attachment.

Each of them sat at their own table and carried on a heated conversation at volumes sufficient to be heard in the lobby at the other end of the building.

"Look at these floors. They haven't touched them in days." I thought I was the only one that noticed that.

"They just don't care."

Well I've been afraid of changing

"Exactly. How long has that dinner roll been under that chair over there?" To be honest, the roll was starting to bother me too. I should have picked it up the day before so that it would be taken care of.

Mom, who hadn't really communicated in any real way in my time there that day, shot me a glare. It was a glare I had not seen since...

And I'm getting older too

I ran a quick internal diagnostic to recall what I may have done to deserve that glare.

Zip.

Nada.

It finally dawned on me that the glare was not directed at me. Something else had gotten enough of Mom's attention that she had to address it. This meant that Mom was having a good day, cognitively speaking.

"Something needs to be done." Linda and Gwendolyn continued to commiserate.

Well, I've been afraid of changing

Mom mouthed something to me.

"I'm sorry. What?" I ask her to repeat it. I didn't initially expect her to remember what she had just said, but Mom surprised me and said it again, just a little bit louder.

I still couldn't hear her.

"I'm sorry Mom, I still didn't hear you. Can you say it again?"

Mom obliged me with a little more volume that only I could hear.

"That lady is crazy."

*I have just about had it up to **here** with her.*

The only time she's not complaining is when she's being nice to the nurses because she needs something. Otherwise, it's just gripe, gripe, gripe all the time. 'Oh I have had a busy day today, delivering the mail and putting all the little gift bags together'.

Give me a break.

Why is she bringing mail to my room? That is NONE of her business! I thought you set it up for all my mail to come to your house. And why is she putting decorations on my door? Isn't the wreath you hung enough?

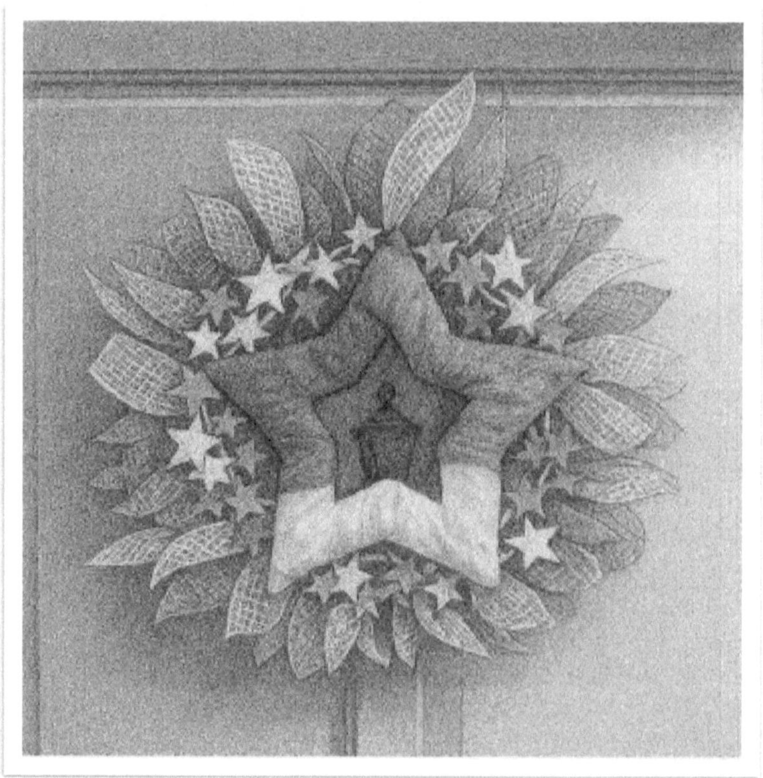

She still owes me $5 for what happened to that guy down the hall the other day. I called it, but she won't admit that I was right.

I would LOVE to go over there and just SMACK her in the mouth.

I held back the urge to break the sound barrier with a guffaw. I also held back the urge to report Mom's assessment about Linda in the group text I had with Wifey and Thumper. That could wait until later.

This was awesome.

Of everything Mom was enduring right now, between the cognitive decline, the inability to move her arms or legs, my excessive uses of malapropisms, the complete dependency on others to take care of her daily activities, and the fact that for all tents and porpoises I had dumped her in a home (my own personal hangup about this whole situation), Linda, the President of the Residents who lived across the hall from room 209 was Mom's biggest irritant.

I responded. "No kidding? Well she's set the bar high for you then, huh?"

And if you see my reflection in the snow-covered hills

Well, the landslide will bring you down

Mom smirked.

<u>**The Non-Mom Favorite**</u>

My office is walking distance from Los Prados Verdes Center for Nursing & Rehabilitation.

Granted, everything is walking distance from a given destination if you have enough time.

Once August 32nd arrived and Mom was now covered by a new insurance company with contracted providers in Texas, the hospital over on the other side of town which had housed her for the last two weeks dispatched us to the right side of town for long term care.

With Mom in a new and closer location, I was able to see her after work every day without fighting cross-town traffic, which just happens to be the bane of my existence.

The first resident I encountered at Prados Verdes was sitting outside the front door the first time I arrived. He donned a t-shirt purchased in a gift shop located at the airport of some vacation destination, a pair of shorts, and socks. His legs were under-developed and jutted straight out instead of being bent at the knee.

If I had to guess, this guy was sitting outside doing reconnaissance for Linda in service to one of her grand schemes. After all, it never hurts for the President of the Residents to know the arrival and departure schedules of the big wigs from corporate, residents who leave for appointments, vacuum cleaner salesmen, and the smattering of choirs, bands, and orchestras from local schools.

"How ya doin'?" I greeted him as I approached the door.

He just frowned at me, so I moved on. Apparently this resident wasn't familiar with the greeting etiquette we use here in Texas.

Over the following weeks, I continued to encounter him throughout the whole building. This only made sense because he was in room 210, which was just across the hall from Mom.

I continued to greet him whenever I saw him, and he eventually began acknowledging my presence.

By then, I knew his name. I had heard plenty members of staff address him, and he even had a customized highway sign on his door which featured his name. Even though I knew his name, I wasn't going to address him with it until he gave me permission to do so.

One day Mom and I were sitting in the dining room attempting to consume some pureed concoction which found its genetic building blocks in tuna fish salad.

The volume of the music overhead was a little high. I always wondered if that was by design so that the staff working the dining room wouldn't have to field the complaints they couldn't hear.

> *It's knowin' that your door is always open*
>
> *And your path is free to walk*

"Ugh this is tuna." Linda called out to the nurse in charge that night. "Hey Jessica, can I get a grilled cheese sandwich? Gwendolyn do you want one?" Linda and Gwendolyn were the only residents in the dining room with the presence of mind to reject what was on the menu in favor of a sandwich.

And it's knowing I'm not shackled

By forgotten words and bonds

My sentiments exactly. I've never been a fan of seafood, and the smell of tuna fish didn't set well with me. Mom used to make it all the time when I was young, and it always went best on white Wonder bread with Ruffles potato chips on the side. Honestly, I don't think I've had that stuff since I was a teenager.

I've always appreciated that Wifey's iodine allergy kept her from eating or preparing seafood. No more tuna fish, or any other fish.

Or something that somebody said

Because they thought we fit together walkin'

Nurse Jessica's attention was on someone else which kept her from prioritizing the sandwich order. "Ellen don't leave yet. You need to eat some more so your blood sugar stays up."

"Okay." Ellen had pulled away from her table which was next to ours and was preparing for a takeoff. Since Jessica had disrupted her initial escape attempt, Ellen turned her chair around and bellied her well-dressed 80 lb. frame back up to her dinner.

By the rivers of my memory

And for hours you're just gentle on my mind

Anthony, one of the C.N.A.'s was seated at a separate table with Doc Brown on his right and Mr. OK on his left. Doc Brown continued to talk up a storm at amazing velocity. Whenever she reduced her speed to just below 88 mph to take a breath, Anthony would introduce a spoonful of tuna fish into her flux capacitor. He would then switch his attention to Mr. OK and offer him a bite. To which, Mr. OK would agree with great volume. "**OKAAAAY**."

Out of the corner of my eye, I could see Ellen gesticulating wildly to the other side of the dining room, as if she were trying to get the attention of Mom's neighbor from the across the hall using her own customized version of seasoned citizen semaphore.

It seemed to have worked because he looked over in Ellen's direction.

Once eye contact was established, Ellen tugged each of her ears, held three fingers to her chin and then clapped twice.

What's going on with Ellen? It looks like she's coaching 3^(rd) base and calling for a bunt.

> *I still might run in silence, tears of joy might stain my face*

> *And the summer sun might burn me 'til I'm blind*

From the far side of the dining room, Mom's neighbor from room 210 started coughing. As his esophagus continued desperately to negotiate the tuna fish on a deliberate mission to fail miserably, his shaved head cast brilliant shades of red, like the vermillion hue of the 1992 Mercury Topaz that Wifey drove when we first met, accented with just hints of the blood of angry men from the French revolution. All three members of staff and the rest of us who were cognizant of what was going on focused our attention on our friend to determine if someone was having an episode or just needed to chew his food better.

Ellen looked around to verify that no one was paying attention to her and exploited the distraction. By the time I turned my head in her direction, she was scuttling her way right out of there as fast as she could, bound for her room.

> *I dip my cup of soup back from a gurglin'*

> *Cracklin' caldron in some train yard*

Tasha, one of the other C.N.A.'s working the room that night addressed the coughing. "Don't make me come over there and give you CPR. You won't want that."

The coughing stopped and Ellen was gone. Who would have thought the residents were coordinating distractions like this?

I just realized something. You're going to write about this aren't you?

—Yup. There are some things you just can't make up.

Right now, the best story I have involves a roller-disco flashmob at an outdoor mall, led by a muse belting out Xanadu. The whole spectacle's just a diversion while a crew knocks over a jewelry store to steal the Gene Kelly diamond. Naturally, a dragon who is later revealed to be in cahoots with the muse crashes the scene. Just when you think the twists are done, you learn the muse is a gnarly, haggard-lookin' succubus —and nobody notices, because her very distinct scent blinds everyone to reality. That scent, of course, is the scent of rainbows.

Randy where do you get this stuff?

—Well that storyline comes from your love of the movie Xanadu and my hatred of flashmobs.

Even still, what we're seeing here is a lot better.

The dining resumed, and I continued to spoon feed Mom.

This stuff isn't as good as the tuna fish I used to make.

Quit making that face Randy. You used to eat my tuna fish all the time. Besides, you don't even have to eat it right now.

—A, it smells bad, and 2, there aren't enough Ruffles in the world to ever get me to eat that stuff again.

> *That you're waitin' from the backroads*
>
> *By the rivers of my memories*

As the other residents finished their dinner, they filed out of the dining room one by one. Mom was slow to eat, so we were usually among the last ones to leave.

Once Mom dispatched the last of her tuna fish, I fed her some pureed cake that smelled just sweet enough to give my olfactory nerve a cavity. My un-named friend who just twenty minutes earlier had come perilously close to receiving a superfluous Heimlich maneuver from a cute C.N.A. approached our table on his way out.

"How are you doing sir?" He called me "sir".

"We're doing good, how are you?"

Mom shot me a look that only I could understand. *Gimme another bite of that cake.*

"Oh I'm doing good. Hey, my name is Martin."

And there was the name, and I had permission to use it.

Throughout our time at Prados Verdes, I saw Martin about as often as I saw Mom. He would share stories about his parents and siblings with me all the time.

Of all the residents and staff that I got to know there, Martin was my non-Mom favorite.

Easel Painting As A Projective Technique

And then there was Ruth.

I'm certain that if Ruth had been in that dining room complaining about the service and how the administration at Los Prados Verdes Center for Nursing & Rehabilitation just didn't care, Mom would have had the same reaction that she did to the President of the Residents.

Don't doubt me on this.

Ruth had a way of assuming the role of tour guide wherever she went and would point out the most obvious and inane things that could be pointed out.

Once she was retired, Ruth would frequently audit courses at the local university and made several trips abroad to take a summer course or two at Oxford University.

Ruth spent the better part of her professional life teaching grade school in west Texas. In the process, she developed long lasting relationships with a lot of her students while ignoring the relationships with her immediate family.

Of course she didn't see it that way, but there was plenty of evidence from her sister, her father, and her only daughter that suggested otherwise.

When Ruth was nineteen, her mother Ruby died on the day before her 47th birthday. Ruby had breast cancer, and a surgical intervention left her with the infection that took her life.

A few years later, Ruth met the man she called Butch at the altar at a Methodist church in Tahoka, Texas.

Initially their attempts to start a family failed.

After three years of trying, Butch and Ruth welcomed a daughter.

A year and a half later, triplets arrived just before Christmas.

Carol Jane passed on Christmas day when she was just 2 days old.

Peggy June passed a week later.

A few months later, on March 2, Martha Jean passed.

By then, Ruth and Butch were done trying to have additional kids and focused on their careers and their daughter instead.

They endeavored to raise a genius while working as teachers.

In fact, when Ruth wrote her master's thesis on analyzing the intelligence quotient of young children via their finger painting, her daughter was prominently featured as one of the test subjects. It should go without saying that <u>An Experimental Study of Easel Painting As A Projective Technique With Nursery School Children</u> was dedicated to her daughter as well.

Another tragic event was just around the corner.

There was a polio outbreak in west Texas around the time the little girl was five, and she contracted it. Again, Ruth and Butch were devastated. After all those years trying to have children, coupled with the loss of Carol Jane, Peggy June, and Martha Jean, they were afraid they were going to lose their only daughter.

Ruth and Butch prepared themselves for the worst when they had to put their only daughter in the hospital. This left their little girl with lifelong feelings of abandonment.

The relationship between Ruth, Butch, and their daughter was never the same after that.

Ruth and Butch expected perfection in their daughter and even sent her straight to first grade as a 5-year-old. After all, if you're going to raise a genius, don't bother sending your child to Kindergarten.

The years progressed and Ruth, more than Butch, became the source of pain and anguish within her daughter. Ruth realized this but never showed it. Instead, she directed the finger-painting, Kindergarten-skipping genius of a daughter of hers into a course of study which would put her on a path guaranteed to help her realize her full potential.

After graduating college with a degree in Library Sciences and the complicated mathematics involved with the Dewey Decimal System, Ruth's daughter met a guy, got married, and started her own family. When the opportunity came up to leave west Texas and the underside of Ruth's thumb, her daughter jumped at the chance to do so.

Butch retired a few years later and spent his retirement harvesting pecans from the trees in his yard. Ruth, who was 11 years younger, continued to work as a teacher until she retired.

After retiring, Ruth pursued mentoring others with realizing their full potential. She volunteered her skills as a teacher to help adults who were trying to make a better life for themselves. On many an occasion, she would even anonymously pay their tuition at the local college.

For what it's worth, I never encountered Ruth in the traditional sense at Los Prados Verdes Center for Nursing & Rehabilitation.

I didn't see her in the lobby when I checked in to see Mom.

I didn't see her walking around in the hallways.

She was never in the dining room.

She was there though.

Ruth was there because Mom was her daughter.

Ruth was there in Mom's healthy distrust for western medicine and fear of being abandoned in a medical facility. In fact it only occurs to me now that the issue with Mom having polio when she was young fed into her desire to pursue alternative treatment for whatever ails us.

When Thumper and I were teenagers, Mom and Dad divorced.

Dad was transferred back to Texas a year later and took Thumper with him. I stayed with Mom in Wyoming because I was near the end of my time in high school and had no interest in leaving.

Over the following years, Mom and Grandma started reconciling some of their differences. The two of them got along famously provided there was a thousand miles between them that could only be connected by the occasional handwritten correspondence or long-distance call.

Grandma was always fond of Dad and continued to foster a relationship with him when he got back to Texas. So much so that she named him to take care of her affairs when she rewrote her Will. It was understandable at the time, as Dad was in Texas and geographically close enough to address any issues which could come up. Taking care of Ruth's affairs was the last thing Mom would want to do, but at the same time, she didn't appreciate that the role would fall to her ex-husband.

So much for reconciliation.

On a side note, when I make reference to Grandma "re-writing her Will", I mean she "wrote" it. She had taken a course at the local college on Englitch to Legalese / Legalese to Englitch and decided that when she needed to re-do her estate planning, she didn't need to pay a lawyer to draw up the appropriate documents.

Instead, she "wrote" her Last Will and Testament down using all those fancy italicized phrases like *'per stirpes'*, *'animus revocandi,'* and *'canis meus id comedit'* on lined notebook paper (college ruled). She then kidnapped a couple of her neighbors to the office of the local notary public so that they could witness her signing her holographic Will.

Nothing says you've lived up to your full potential until you've handwritten your own Will.

But I digress.

Tensions between Mom and Grandma got worserer.

When Wifey and I got married, we underwent all the traditional rituals a wedding party executes for such a blessed event. In addition to the axe throwing demonstrations and primer on knife fighting, we had a rehearsal at the church and then adjourned to the all-you-can-eat buffet on the other side of the freeway for a rehearsal dinner.

Thumper and I used to hit that place all the time when we first moved to town.

Grandma had been invited to all the festivities. From the rehearsal activities on the night before to the wedding the next day, she was welcome and encouraged to come.

Grandma opted not to attend the wedding for two reasons, one of which was fully understandable.

By then, Grandpa (Butch) was in a nursing home in San Angelo, and Grandma was concerned about leaving him. Underneath the plausible reason for not coming, we all knew deep down that Grandma didn't want to get caught up in moments of intense fellowship with Mom on my wedding day.

Mom had planned to attend our wedding and then stay in town a few days. She was still living in Wyoming at the time and had driven down to San Antonio with Ginger in tow.

Ginger was an 11-year-old German Shepherd / Husky mix and was going to be living with us until Thumper could find a place to live where he could have a dog.

After staying in San Antonio for a few days, Mom would head back home, but not before making an obligatory stop in San Angelo to see her parents.

On the night we got hitched, Wifey and I took a quick trip out of town to hone our new axe throwing and knife fighting skills for a few days.

Upon returning home, Dad was there and hit me with some news.

"Randy, your Grandfather passed away last Friday."

"Friday? The day before the wedding? Why are we only learning this now?"

"Well Ruth didn't want his passing to ruin your wedding."

Furthermore, it turns out that Grandma didn't even let Mom know about it either. She was waiting for Mom to arrive in San Angelo before delivering the news in person that Butch, her husband, Mom's father, and my Grandfather had passed away.

Okay, Grandma didn't want to spoil the wedding by delivering bad news the day before.

Fine.

Certainly, it was understandable that she wanted to tell Mom in person, but that was the wrong option.

If she could pick up a phone and notify Dad, why didn't she just track down Mom instead of putting Dad in a precarious Kobayashi Maru where he had to navigate the more comfortable position between a rock and a hard place?

For the uninitiated, Kobayashi Maru is a no-win scenario which was an underlying theme in a popular science fiction movie about forty years ago. The same theme re-appeared when the series of popular movies was rebooted with a new cast, more advanced special effects, and other technical pizzazz.

High tensions between Mom and Grandma were now a goal compared to what was about to happen. Thumper and I made the call immediately to make sure Mom was aware of what had happened, so later that day, on the day before she was slated to drive to San Angelo, we told her.

Naturally, Mom was upset about the passing of her father. After all, she had a better relationship with Butch. Mom's anger was obviously compounded by Grandma's attempted orchestration of how the news would be delivered several days after Butch's passing.

On the other side of the issue, there was Grandma. Naturally, we had to let her know that we had told Mom. When Grandma learned this, she was not happy.

Again, I'll make a reference to the aforementioned "precarious Kobayashi Maru where one has to navigate the more comfortable position between a rock and a hard place."

"What if on her trip out there, Mom had gone directly to the nursing home to see Grandpa before seeing you?" I asked her. "She would have gotten the news from some stranger at the nursing home instead of a family member." Beloved or otherwise.

After hearing the issue from a different point of view, Grandma was relieved to know that we had told Mom about what had happened.

On a side note, three of her favorite singers, my dog, and the Queen of England passed away in the time Mom was under my care, and I didn't let any members of staff pass that news on to her either. That was my job, however I don't think she really cared about Betty as much as she did about Olivia, Christine, Loretta, or Faith.

Mom did stop in San Angelo on her way back home, and a heated discussion ensued. I never got an update from Mom or Grandma on what exactly transpired in that interaction, but I'm pretty sure that was the last communication Mom would have with Grandma.

Grandma passed away a little over a year later in a car accident.

Dining Room Orders

Mr. OK had full use of his arms.

He would have had full use of his legs if they were still intact.

When Mom first took on her assigned duties in room 209 of Los Prados Verdes Center for Nursing & Rehabilitation, Linda, the President of the Residents lived across the hall from her.

Mr. OK was stationed a few rooms down the hall.

This was problematic on the weekends when most of the immobile residents remained restricted to quarters. There were many a time on those weekends where Mr. OK would use his limited ability to express himself when trying to get the attention of the nursing staff.

"**OKAAAAY.**

OKAAAAY....."

If it ever bothered Mom, she never showed it.

Linda couldn't stand it.

So much so, that the President of the Residents exercised her authority, clout, and various bits of dirt she had on the staff to get herself relocated down the hall and out of earshot from one of her less than articulate neighbors.

"OKAAAAY."

I became curious about what Mr. OK did before coming to Prados Verdes. Even though I made eye contact with him many a time and even said "Hello" a few times, he never really accepted my attempts at conversation.

At one point I asked Carolina, one of the C.N.A.'s about him. "Hey, what did Mr. OK do in his previous life? Was he military or law enforcement or something along that line?"

"He yelled a lot."

"OKAAAAY."

One night in the dining room, Mr. OK was in rare form.

It was just before serving time, and most of the residents had already arrived and were waiting for their vittles.

As always, music played overhead, however the genre choice didn't really seem to be appropriate for this crowd. It was better suited for my generation instead. I'm guessing the 20-something charged with selecting the station was told to choose something old but didn't pick something that was quite old enough.

Ellen was at a table nearby talking about going home next weekend.

Minnie and Rosa were seated at the table they normally shared.

Martin had just arrived and was looking out the bay window next to his table.

Linda and Gwendolyn were talking about the high stakes bingo game scheduled for later.

Mr. OK was at his normal table. His normal table partner Doc Brown wasn't in the dining room that night. Instead, a new resident was seated there with Mr. OK in her wheelchair with her head tilted down.

"Okay Miss Betty. If the plate is a clock, the lasagna is at 2 o'clock, the broccoli is at 6 o'clock, and there's a dinner roll at 10 o'clock". Miss Betty was blind and needed a description of whatever was being served up to her for consumption.

That's great it starts with an earthquake

Birds and snakes and aeroplanes

It's unfortunate that Doc Brown chose to go on a mission to fix the timeline instead of going to the dining room that night. Mr. OK was unusually talkative and barking orders to all the bit players in whatever hallucination he was either participating in or directing.

If Doc Brown and her perpetual flux capacitor had been there to interact in such a conversation, it would have been a glorious cacophony.

Alas, Doc Brown wasn't there, so it was just Mr. OK loudly delivering very direct and transparent instructions to Miss Betty in a one-way conversation.

Or so I thought.

"OKAAY people, we've gotten an update from a well-placed source that inspectors from the state are coming in next week. The time to act is now if we're going to be taken seriously. Is that clear?"

"Yes."

Wait. What?

Betty had responded to Mr. OK.

Her head was still tilted down, but she was going to take an active role in Mr. OK's dictates to the troops.

Six o'clock TV hour

Don't get caught in foreign tower

Slash and burn return

Listen to yourself churn

"I didn't hear you."

Betty raised her voice a little. "Yes sir!"

"That's better. Now I need you all to get all your loose ends resolved because not everybody is coming back. Report to Minnie over there to get your assignments. For those of you on lookout, be sure to provide regular status updates to room 209.

—Huh?

Mom shot me a glare. *Hush.*

"When the time comes, everyone who doesn't have an assignment needs to gather every extra wheelchair, walker, bedpan, medicine cart, Hoyer Lift, and portable toilet seat they can to build a barricade across the south wall of this room. Now repeat that back to me."

"Gather anything we can to build a barricade across the south wall."

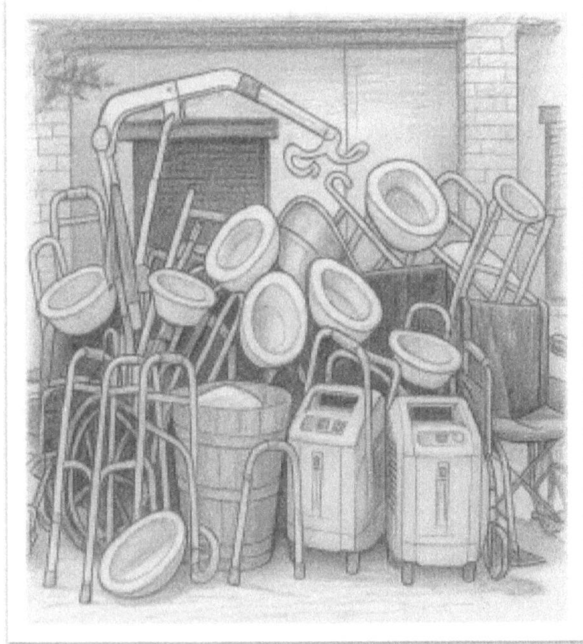

Mr. OK continued. **"Make sure those of us who need oxygen have working machines where the tubes are not crimped and they're in good working order."**

"Check the oxygen machines."

"We're also going to need resources on the inside to help us with our daily needs once we gain control. After all, not every patriot can dress or feed themselves."

"Find some nurses who will help us."

"I want you to muster the troops here in the dining room at oh-eight-hundred tomorrow and await further instructions."

"Mustard the troops tomorrow at oh-eight-hundred. Yes sir."

"One more thing. Find the person who put that infernal racket on the speakers for dinner tonight. They'll be the first against the wall once we take over."

Minnie nodded and shot me a menacing glare.

The other night I tripped a nice

Continental drift divide

Mountains sit in a line

Before the remaining battle plans could be delivered and acknowledged, Mr. OK got his dinner tray and discontinued his leadership.

When Mom's dinner arrived, she rolled her eyes a little.

It's the end of the world as we know it

It's the end of the world as we know it

Mom looked a little different than she had in recent weeks. It was as if she wasn't completely up to snuff. "You doin' all right Mom?"

I feel fine.

Mom didn't want to eat.

Her lack of appetite wasn't completely uncommon. Usually at least once a week she showed a lack of interest in eating dinner. I could only guess why.

Actually I don't feel fine. In fact, I'm getting a headache and I'm chilly.

Tonight was different though. Her attitude seemed to be a little more lethargic and a little less stubborn.

Oh, I'm not feeling good. Take me to my room.

Something was different.

Come on, let's go.

I tried a few more times to feed her some lasagna, which was positioned at a quarter past 2 o'clock on her plate as it was oriented in front of her.

"It doesn't seem like you're very hungry Mom. Do you want to go back to your room?"

She flashed a look of acceptance on her face and nodded slightly. *Yes.*

"Okay, let's go."

On the way back to Mom's room, we encountered Ellen. This was interesting, because I thought I had just seen her in the dining room moments before.

Ellen was an expert at the practice of dine and dash, so she must have skipped out on her check shortly after her lasagna arrived.

"Hi Ellen."

Ellen's muscle memory took over.

In one fluid motion, she took her glasses off and wrapped the ends of the purple beaded chain around each of her hands, leaving the longer piece in the middle ready to wrap around the neck of anyone who got too close to the truth.

Ellen cocked her head up and squinted a bit to see who was talking to her. Once she realized it was me, she positioned the garrote garnished glasses back on her face. "Oh hi sweetheart."

Mom rolled her eyes. *You have her fooled, don't you?*

Just by coincidence, Teresita, the C.N.A. who was taking care of Mom that day was in room 209 straightening up when we arrived. "How did Miss Barb do with dinner tonight?"

The C.N.A.'s usually asked me this whenever I fed Mom so that they could update their own records on Mom's progress.

"Barely 10%. Something is different about her tonight."

Teresita felt Mom's forehead. "She has a fever. She may not be feeling well."

Duh.

"When you say fever, do mean she may have Covid?"

"Well it's going around right now."

"Yeah I keep getting emails about it from upper management."

"We'll test her and let you know the results."

<u>Living In The Age Of Covid</u>

Subject Covid-19 Notification

From   Mgmt – Los Prados Verdes Center for Nursing & Rehabilitation

To   Los Prados Verdes Family

Sent   Friday, December 30, 2022, 5:33 P.M.

Good evening Prados Verdes Family,

We wanted to inform you that we have had five patients test positive for Covid-19 in the last 24 hours. About a third of our current positive patients will be coming off isolation tomorrow and are doing well. We continue to follow all state, local, and federal guidelines. Please stay safe and let me know if you have any questions. Thank you for your continued support and prayers.

Kind Regards,

Los Prados Verdes Center for Nursing & Rehabilitation

The information contained in this transmission may contain privileged and confidential information, including patient information protected by federal and state privacy laws. It is intended only for the use of the person(s) named above. If you are not the intended recipient, you are hereby notified that any review, dissemination, distribution, or duplication of this communication is strictly prohibited. If you are not the intended recipient, please contact the sender by reply email and destroy all copies of the original message and any attachments.

107

Blossom

My brother and I love our dogs.

Thumper has Maggie, a little white dog which breaches post-Labor Day dress code etiquette and sports an italicized French name for her breed. I won't try to lay down an assault on the language by trying to pronounce or spell it out, because the only French words I know are "fry", "dip", and "Coton de Tulear".

Every time Thumper ever came into town to brunch with Mom, he would bring Maggie along for the ride. Mom seemed to enjoy that.

One of the reasons we love our dogs is because it was ingrained in our little skulls via Mom's love for Dodger, our childhood pet.

Dodger was born about a year before me. As I understand it, Mom and Dad had gone to see his Uncle Roy.

It occurs to me that everyone should have an Uncle named Roy.

Dodger just happened to be one of the newest members of the household as part of a litter of puppies which had been born to the family dog.

Uncle Roy had talked up the possibility of Mom and Dad taking one of the puppies. Mom and Dad were non-committal at that time. Mom never had a dog as a pet growing up because her mother was either afraid of them or didn't like them.

As Mom and Dad arrived, Uncle Roy admonished the puppies that company was present and to show some respect and hospitality.

The Artful Dodger (as named by Roy's daughters and Dad's cousins) got the signal loud and clear, ran up to Mom and Dad, and piddled right there on the floor.

It was love at first sight.

That summer day in 1982 when he passed away was my first real encounter with losing a loved one.

Years later, Wifey and I were looking to make Christmas a little easier on the wallet and decided to get a dog for the family instead of buying a whole bunch of gifts.

One night we went over to the Humane Society to see if we could find a new friend to adopt. After wandering around a while, we happened upon a little black and white puppy who looked like the product of a chance meeting between a Labrador and a non-Labrador.

The sign on the kennel said "Buddy".

When the volunteer brought Buddy to us outside in the 'Get To Know You' yard, he approached Juniorette and piddled on the ground right in front of her.

We were ready to take him home.

The problem was that it was closing time, and there wasn't enough time to process the adoption before the doors were locked.

The kids and I would return the next morning for Buddy. Wifey had to work that morning and couldn't join us.

Of course we weren't aware of the other family who was there at the same time. They also wanted to adopt Buddy.

I became aware of that the next morning when we arrived at opening time. I was polite enough to hold the door open for the family who got in there first. They called dibs on the dog before we could.

So the kids and I took another look around, each going our separate ways.

On my own little tour of the facility, I happened upon a kennel with two puppies. Their name tags said 'Blossom' and 'Buttercup'. As I stared at those two, I couldn't help but think that I was looking at a few of Buddy's littermates.

It turns out I was.

A few hours later Wifey got home from work and was introduced to Blossom. We then proceeded with a renaming ceremony.

My suggestion of Goofball was roundly rejected in favor of Faith.

Over the years, Faith continued to amaze and inspire us with her brilliant displays of jumping on the kitchen counters during thunderstorms, offering up recently deceased squirrels to Wifey, and liberating the property of the evil spirits which possess bedding plants, window screens, and garden hoses.

During the lockdown when I had to work from home and Faith was already considered to be an old lady, she would go on walks with me during my breaks and lunches. Even then, that little treadmill not only helped me increase my step count, but she also provided resistance training with sudden lunges in all directions other than straightforward.

By the time Mom came to live with us, Faith was nearly sixteen, and not as concerned about thunderstorms, squirrels, or evil spirits in the flora and fauna out in the yard. Even still, she was joining me on walks, just without the resistance training she gave in her youth. By then, Charlie the Silver Lab had joined us, so I was walking two dogs at once.

Those two dogs and I had an unspoken agreement on who was in charge on those walks.

Granted, I was the one picking up their gastronomical indiscretions.

Aside from those walks, Faith had spent a better part of her day for the last three years on our bed. Faith was just a month younger than Mom's late dog Brandi. A month after her birthday, Faith developed what I thought was an abscess just above her upper left canine. The vet disagreed and characterized it as a malignant tumor that couldn't be removed.

We all agreed at the time that Faith still had some gumption and would happily tell Charlie to get off her lawn. We took no action at the time.

As the months went on, the tumor started to reduce in size. At the same time, Faith would have difficulty eating. Wifey and I began hand feeding her soft food which she sometimes ate. On all those other occasions, she sent it back and referred to it as "low-grade dog food".

One day, while sitting on a five-gallon bucket trying to get her to eat, I went a little dark. "Geez, it's like my life is filled with feeding ole ladies. This one here, and one over at the nursing home."

In all honesty, Mom would have liked that one. After all, one of her friends had characterized Mom's sense of humor as "wicked".

In March, we took Faith for her semi-annual exam at the vet. Strange enough, the vet could no longer feel the tumor in her mouth. Again, we all agreed that it wasn't time to say goodbye to Faith yet.

A month later, I arrived home from a long day at work, followed by a few hours with Mom and all my other friends at Los Prados Verdes Center for Nursing & Rehabilitation.

Back at home, when I sat down to eat my own dinner, I was surprised to see that Faith had left the comfort of the master bedroom and had decided to join Charlie and me at the dinner table. One of us was seated on the bench, reading an electronic book, and eating a drumstick of the chicken varietal. The other two of us were seated on the floor, maintaining strict, unwavering eye contact with each bite. The chicken was not being shared as much as originally anticipated.

Faith hadn't begged at the dinner table like that in months.

The next morning, I got up like I do every Wednesday and got ready for work. Wifey had fallen asleep in her recliner out in the living room, so Faith had appropriated Wifey's side of the bed as her own. Once I was dressed, I would get Faith up and get her fed before heading to work in Mom's low-mileage,, 2011 Subaru Outback.

As I approached the bed to wake her up, I found Faith's head to be tucked a little too far into her chest than what she would consider comfortable.

Her stomach wasn't moving up and down to show me she was breathing..

Faith had passed away, quietly in her sleep sometime last night.

That one hit hard.

Five years ago, we had to say goodbye to our pit bull Hope when she developed bone cancer. That one also hit hard because of how quickly it happened. Hope started showing signs of it in March and was gone a month later.

With Faith, we knew it was coming.

We just didn't know when.

We knew between her age and her condition, that it was a matter of days, weeks, or months before she would pass away.

On a Wednesday morning, on April 26th, I sat on the backyard porch with tears in my eyes.

Nine months ago, Mom's little cocker spaniel passed away. I know that Mom was upset about Brandi's passing. I know this because I know how much she loved her dogs.

I also know that Mom was fond of Faith. In recent years when Mom had come to Texas for a visit, those two old ladies got along famously. Faith could have been Mom's dog as easily as Brandi was.

I didn't expect Mom would be able to show any sort of emotion over the passing of Faith. After all, Mom was in a progressive decline and not really registering anything as much as she was last fall. Deep down, I knew there would be a part of her that would mourn the loss though.

As I walked through the door to room 209 that afternoon, Mom was sitting in her wheelchair watching TV. I pulled up a chair and sat next to her.

"I'm afraid I have some sad news, Mom."

The look she gave me showed a certain level of concern.

I called up a picture of Faith on my phone and showed it to her. "Our little dog Faith passed away this morning." It was still hard to say that aloud.

Mom looked at the picture and then at me. *Oh, I'm sorry to hear that, Randy. I sure did like her.*

Mom didn't say anything, nor did I expect her to.

Mom didn't show any emotion, short of staring at the picture of Faith. *She was such a good little dog.*

"I sure am going to miss that dog. Of all the dogs we've ever had, starting with Dodger, we had her the longest."

I guess you have one less ole lady to feed now.

—Yeah I guess I do.

Flash

———

As a short kid, I had a diminutive strike zone.

Sure Jose Altuve has one too, but he doesn't draw the walks that I did in my youth.

On a hot Wyoming day in the middle of May when that red goo they put in thermometers may have risen beyond 80 degrees, I exploited that strike zone to get on base during what may or may not have been a big game.

It's been a while, and I only remember one specific detail from that game, so bear with me.

As I stood there on base taking the occasional lead-off, I put things on autopilot. I didn't know the count, or even how many outs there were.

The coach then barked an order at me. "Okay Randy, on the next pitch, no matter whether it's a ball or a strike, go to 2nd base."

"Got it." I was ready to go. I was about to commit an audacious act of grand theft base.

The pitcher began his motion, reared back, and hurled the ball at the plate. Once I saw the ball cross the plate, I bolted.

"Juuuuuuuuuust a bit outside," Bob Uecker announced as I arrived at my destination.

I didn't have to slide or dive. The catcher didn't try to burn one down there to throw me out. "How 'bout that?" I thought to myself. "Neckless fireplugs, can actually run."

The voice of Dad rang out from the stands. "Way to go Flash!"

As I collected myself from such a harrowing 60-foot run, I reassessed the situation.

A new batter was coming up to the plate and the kid that was just batting was now on first base.

And then the epiphany struck.

I didn't need to bolt as if I was stealing the base.

There were two outs, and that kid had a full count. If he drew a walk, I was going to 2nd base anyway. If he struck out, the inning was over. If he hit the ball, I had to get to 2nd base before getting caught up in a force out.

More importantly, I had just been ascribed a new moniker that wasn't as disparaging as the other nicknames I had accrued over the years.

The name of Flash stuck for the rest of the school year. Of all the nicknames a short fat kid could endure in his youth, that one was charitable. It didn't matter that the name was equated with my lack of situational awareness on the baseball diamond. It didn't even mean that I was fast because I wasn't. We've already established the fact that fire plugs with no necks shouldn't run.

Many years later when I was coaching Junior, Dad came to town to watch a game. At one point, while I was sitting on my 5-gallon bucket, working the scorebook, calling off the batting order, and avoiding the smells that 11 and 12-year-old boys emit in a dugout, Dad yelled out at me from the stands. "Hey Flash!"

This last year, the end of May arrived none too soon.

We were busy during that time with a trip to Dallas to celebrate the first birthday of our grandson. A few days after we returned from that trip our grandson arrived with his parents to make the rounds with family in the area. In essence, we went there and then they came here.

This gave Mom a chance to see her great grandson a second time.

By then, a year had passed since she last saw him. There had been an opportunity several months before when the kid was in town for the holidays.

Convincing him and his parents to visit Prados Verdes where Mom and several of her compatriots were being isolated in a hot zone with Covid was understandably a non-starter.

Given her mental state, I've got to wonder what Mom thought of seeing the toddler and adult versions of her oldest son at the same time.

He's a cute kid, Randy. Too bad he looks like you.

—Yeah, I've been apologizing to his mother about that.

A few days later, Thumper came to town to celebrate Mom's birthday.

Afterward, we all returned to our normal schedules.

Various Tharps returned to the Dallas area, and other Tharps stayed here at home.

Mom's schedule returned to a sense of normalcy as well. If she were dressed and ready when I got there after work, I would take her for a stroll outside in the parking lot. Each time we did that, I pointed out a certain low-mileage, 2011 Subaru Outback which was parked in the same place every day.

After the walk, we would go for whatever fresh, pureed vittles and frenetic chatter the staff and residents of Los Prados Verdes Center for Nursing & Rehabilitation had to offer.

In the following weeks, things started to change.

Mom began eating less of her dinner, and she was sleeping more. There was one night when we were waiting in the dining room for dinner to arrive that she dozed off right there at the table. Even the dictates and proclamations emanating from the President of the Residents failed to phase Mom or keep her from taking a nap.

I shared my concerns with Bobbie, one of the nurses who was taking care of Mom, to see if she or others had noticed similar behavior during the parts of the day when I wasn't there.

They had.

June progressed, and the decline continued.

Juneteenth arrived just as expected.

In June, it was right after the eighteenth, and just before the twentieth.

I'm given to understand that word of Lincoln's Emancipation Proclamation arrived in Texas on June 19, 1860-somthin'.

Having learned about Wyoming history in my formative years, I don't have all the details beyond the knowledge I just dropped up above.

Irregardlessly, the date and its abbreviated name was made a federal holiday last year.

In my work in the financial services industry, I'm off on federal holidays. This presented me with some extra time off.

I needed a minor recharge.

I had been busy at home, busy at work, and busy with Mom.

Since I had a little time off from the office, I decided to take in an early showing of the movie *The Flash*.

I've never really been an avid comic fan; however I do tend to check out the movies they inspire in hopes of seeing something new. Even still, if I were to designate a favorite comic book character, I would have to say it's Flash.

That goes back to an incident on the baseball field when I was about eleven, but I won't bore you with the details...

Again.

The next day, I was back in the office when a noise emitted by my phone reminded me of the spin cycle on the washing machine at home.

Ooga-Chaka, Ooga-Ooga,

Ooga-Chaka, Ooga-Ooga,

Ooga-Chaka, Ooga-Ooga

"Hooked on a Feeling" is a 1968 pop song written by Mark James and originally performed by B.J. Thomas. Fortunately, my phone was in silent mode. Otherwise the chant which precedes the 1974 Blue Swede version of that song would have broken the silence at work.

Since the phone was set to silent and I had earbuds in my hearing holes, I'm the only one that heard it. My heart sank when I saw the call was coming from Los Prados Verdes Center for Nursing & Rehabilitation. I mentally prepared myself for the call I had feared for the last nine months.

"Hi Randy, it's Bobbie at Prados Verdes." Bobbie's voice tone told me that this wasn't the call I was afraid of. Instead, they wanted to change one of Mom's medications to further enhance her appetite. They needed my permission to do so.

"Ya know I gotta tell you. I get nervous every time I see you people calling."

Bobbie apologized, even though she didn't need to. She then broached a delicate subject. "Does Miss Barbara have a DNR order in place with us?"

A Do Not Resuscitate order, or DNR, is paperwork which provides instructions to healthcare workers to take no action to resuscitate an individual in the event they need it.

"I haven't signed anything, but I know that Mom wouldn't want to be resuscitated in her current condition, especially since it's declining."

"You know, without that order in place, we are required to perform CPR on her if she codes. As small and frail as she is, we're bound to break a rib in the process."

That's all Mom needed now was to code, be resuscitated, only to have to deal with a broken rib.

Yesterday, I saw *The Flash*.

It's a movie about a superhero who could run so fast that he could achieve time travel without the benefit of a Flux Capacitor. Once he discovered that, he opted to travel into the past where he could stop the murder of his mother.

By the third act, after he had tried everything he could to save her, he accepted the fact that his mother's fate was sealed.

My review of the movie boils down to two words.

It resonated.

Eleven months ago, I got a call from Mom. She used her friend Cheryl's phone because she had neglected to charge her own. That explained why I had lost contact with Mom in the days and weeks prior.

"Brandi died."

"Oh Mom, I'm sorry."

You know when Dodger died I was so heart-broken. That's why I was so quick to get Ginger afterward.

And then Chowsky disappeared.

And then Ginger ran away.

And then I had to have Chinook put to sleep.

And then you and Bobby had to say goodbye to Sunny.

And then poor Daisy passed away.

Now, Brandi is gone, and I don't know what I'm going to do. I have no real reason to do anything anymore.

Without saying so much as a word, Mom spoke volumes to me on what she needed.

—Mom, I'm coming to get you.

All the signs I saw in the months leading to that phone call were just the opening crawl on the big screen designed to bring the audience up to speed on what was going on.

To that point, I didn't even know what the milestone would be which would put my plan to get Mom to Texas into motion.

I just knew it when it happened.

Now, eleven months later, Mom was broadcasting a new message. In this case, she was just using Bobbie as a conduit because she knew that Bobbie had seen this situation before and had discussed it with the loved ones of many other residents in the years she had worked at Prados Verdes.

During that call on Tuesday the 20th, I came to terms that we were now moving into the third act where nothing else could be done to improve Mom's health or slow her decline.

Later that afternoon, I signed a DNR order for Mom, and I officially put her into hospice care.

Brunching With Thumper

There's something to be said for long road trips and the desire to get back home.

I don't know exactly what that 'something to be said' actually is.

Irregardlessly, whether I was aware of it or not, the exercise of flying to Colorado so that I could sweep Mom out of her perilous condition by moving her to Texas was changing our lives in real time.

Rest assured, I wasn't aware of it. I didn't (and don't) view it as a hero's journey to get her out of her present situation.

Whoever really considers such an adventure to be carried out in a low-mileage, 2011 Subaru Outback?

I figured Mom would move into our extra bedroom and then resume her life without having to manage it.

I would take care of that part.

I'll pause a moment to reflect on my optimism...

Upon arriving in Dallas last night, my little brother Thumper set us up with the best accommodations a one-bedroom downtown apartment had to offer. Mom took the bed, and Thumper took the couch that I had slept on a few nights ago.

A mattress had been laid on the floor at the front door for the coordinator of the unacknowledged hero's journey.

Any armed marauders who chose to enter the apartment to abscond with Thumper's vast assortment of toaster pastries and microwave noodle cups from the pantry closet just next to the front door were going to have to trip over me first.

I don't remember when I woke up on Sunday morning.

Since this was the first mattress I had slept on in a few days, and I had safely gotten Mom out of the immediate danger I had perceived for the last several months, I slept hard.

If the toaster pastry and noodle cup bandits stopped by to replenish their supply at Thumper's expense, I was not there to inhibit their progress.

My agenda that day was straight-forward.

Verify that the low-mileage, 2011 Subaru Outback had not been deemed to have been inappropriately parked and subsequently towed and inappropriately impounded during the previous evening.

Once I was able to verify the low-mileage, 2011 Subaru Outback was still considered to be appropriately parked, stage two of my mission was in full force and effect.

Get Mom home.

Sure there were a couple of things in the middle of that. Thumper wanted to take us to brunch. More importantly, I wanted to do the one thing I was trying to do back in April when all of this started.

I wanted Mom to meet her new great grandson. He lived here in the Dallas area, and I was going to make sure that Mom met him before we headed home.

And then, I was going to resume the carefree life I had developed in recent years.

I'm trying to remember the last time I had brunch.

That's the thing about being locked into the rigid schedule I keep for myself. I go to bed at the same time every night and wake up at the same time every morning. I eat breakfast, lunch, and dinner at the same time every day.

When I work from home, I walk the dogs at specific times of the day, and when I work from the office, I walk the perimeter of either the inner office or the parking garage at the same times every day.

Douglas Adams once said "Time is an illusion. Brunch doubly so."

―――――

Douglas Adams

―――――

Okay, I expect that he said it more than once, and I may have botched the wording on that one.

Irregardlessly, the practice of brunch dictates that I abandon my daily ritual of lovingly slathering flavored cream cheese onto an Everything Bagel and then consuming it along with a few strips of bacon and washing it all down with juice every morning at 7:30 a.m. (central).

Furthermore, going to brunch demands I forego that noon-time walk with the dogs, a habit I developed during the Covid lockdown. That walk precedes the extraction of a frozen grilled delight I deposited into the ice-box in the garage weeks before while performing meal prep.

Going to brunch is a practice which results in me eating breakfast way too late and lunch way too early.

Such behavior inspires a devil-may-care attitude I don't exercise, and it borders on witchcraft.

Furthermore, it's probably fattening.

Even though going to brunch and then visiting Tharp 2.0 (a name one of my in-laws had ascribed to my new grandson) was going to delay our ability to get on the road bound for home, I opted to cast aside my standard rigidity and let the rest of this trip happen as it was meant to be.

If that meant acting like a heathen for an hour or two and eating brunch, so be it.

After all, the only thing that had gone right on this trip was the only thing that absolutely had to go right on this trip. Every obstacle that I encountered along the way, from the delayed flight, to being dropped at the wrong apartment H, to the defective gas door on the low-mileage, 2011 Subaru Outback, to wandering around downtown Dallas at midnight, to guarding Thumper's stash of toaster pastries and noodle cups had been resolved. In the end, I had Mom exactly where I needed to have her. All the other stuff was on the periphery.

Thumper had engineered the brunch for us and several of his friends. He was coming off a bad year in the middle of the Covid lockdowns and had recently started a new job. Thumper wanted to share his newfound success with those who cheered him on during those troubling times.

Even though brunching with strangers was way outside my comfort zone and the day's objective, I couldn't just ditch out under the guise that I had other things to do.

Mom was in decline, and this would be her last social gathering if you don't count dinner with her fellow co-conspirators at Los Prados Verdes Center for Nursing & Rehabilitation.

Thumper had his own concerns about Mom and wanted to take advantage of the last time she could participate in such a gathering.

I couldn't and wouldn't begrudge him that, irregardlessly of the hurry I thought I was in.

It turns out the cantina which features a beautiful staff member who smells like rainbows and affixes blue contact lenses to her brown eyes was open for brunch that morning. It also turns out that one can (and should) order chile rellenos for brunch.

According to a fast and nasty search on the internet, the chile relleno is a dish in Mexican cuisine that originated in the city of Puebla. In 1858, it was described as a "green chile pepper stuffed with minced meat and coated with eggs".

I know it to be a batter-fried green chile pepper stuffed with either cheese, meat, or chicken, and then covered with either chile con queso, or some sort of red sauce.

Irregardlessly, Mom ordered the chile rellenos that day for brunch. For what it's worth, Mom has ordered chile rellenos every time she ever visited us in Texas over the last 30-somethin' years.

That was a pleasant surprise, knowing that her standing menu was comprised of the ingredients found in mint chocolate chip ice cream.

For the next hour or so, we brunched.

We brunched like we had never brunched before. Given that we don't brunch that much, brunching at such an intensity wasn't hard to do.

As our brunch-time hour lingered out of the breakfast-time hour and into the lunch-time hour, the little voice in my head which nags about staying on schedule started admonishing me that we still needed to see Tharp 2.0 and then get on the road.

In the meantime, Mom had succumbed to the excitement of brunch. So much so that after eating a few bites of her chile rellenos, she dozed off right there in the middle of the cantina.

Thumper and I made arrangements for me to run back to his apartment and pack up the low-mileage, 2011 Subaru Outback for the next leg of our journey. I would then return to the cantina which features a beautiful staff member who smells like rainbows and affixes blue contact lenses to her brown eyes to retrieve Mom, who by then would be well rested from a highly productive brunch.

Once I returned, brunch was wrapped up. Thumper's best friend was helping Mom out of her seat and away from the chile rellenos, and Thumper himself had shouldered Mom's purse. The picture I took of that event with him walking toward me with Mom's turquoise purse comfortably shouldered while Mom stands grinning in the background is featured prominently in room 209 at Los

Prados Verdes Center for Nursing & Rehabilitation. Even though I would take a few more pictures of her in the coming weeks, that picture would be the last one featuring her smiling, and fully engaged in the moment.

As Mom and I packed ourselves into her low-mileage, 2011 Subaru Outback and prepared to bid farewell to the cantina where beautiful, brown-eyed girls with blue contact lenses who smell like rainbows will serve you chile rellenos for brunch, Thumper offered up some words of encouragement.

"I just want to tell you both good luck. We're all counting on you."

The First Three Days Of June

The problem with the Saturday to Sunday crew at Los Prados Verdes Center for Nursing & Rehabilitation is that they never get the immobile residents out of bed with any regularity. This is different from the Monday to Friday crew, who get the residents out of bed daily to streamline the feeding process.

On Monday through Friday, the residents who need assistance with eating are all taken to the dining room, and several members of the staff are there to make sure the residents are eating.

On Saturday and Sunday, members of staff feed the residents one at a time in their own rooms. It's not a very efficient process for getting everyone fed, however it does inhibit the more militant of the residents from passing encrypted messages in support of the upcoming revolt.

Mom's birthday fell on a Saturday this year, and Thumper came into town from Dallas to celebrate the occasion.

My hope had been that Mom would be taken out of bed and put in her wheelchair for her birthday. I had even made the request at the nurses station a few days before. Unfortunately, no one got the memo, so we were relegated to celebrating what we expected to be Mom's last birthday with her in bed.

The last time I spent time with Mom on her birthday was four years ago when I flew to Colorado to take care of some housekeeping items.

Our birthdays are two days apart, so this would be a good opportunity for both of us to celebrate.

Okay, our birthdays are 23 years, 11 months, and 28 days apart, but we use the two-day formula when it comes to celebrating them.

In the weeks leading up to that visit, Mom asked me if I would attend services with her on the Sunday I was there, to which I politely declined.

"Why not?"

"Because there's no singular focus on Jesus with that group."

"They talk about Jesus every once in a while."

"Exactly. There's no singular focus on Him. What are they talking about when they're not preaching the Good News?"

"You know I've always gotten the impression that you think I'm involved with a cult or something. I'm not. These are very spiritual people."

"Mom, I'm not going to attend a service where Jesus isn't the singular focus. What else do you want me to say?" Mom dropped the interrogation with the understanding that we would not come to a meeting of the minds.

While in Colorado for our respective birthday celebrations, we had a few agenda items.

Mom had just sold her house (to my relief) and moved into the Enchanted Springs Apartment Complex. I felt like there may have been some moving related tasks she would need me to complete.

We were also slated to attend a session with the personal trainer she had employed over the last several years. We were then going to top it all off with a visit to the armory where I would be outfitted with the weaponry I would need in a few years to take control of Mom's life.

That's right.

Mom needed a Last Will and Testament so that Thumper and I wouldn't spend years fighting over who had to take possession of all the decorative owls and other knickknackery she had amassed in the last fifty years. She also needed to sign power of attorney documents to give one of us the ability to act on her behalf.

Dad had done his in the previous year at the behest of his wife and my step-mother, so that wasn't an issue.

Since Mom had no estate planning in place, I arranged the birthday visit to help get that part done for her. I've heard too many horror stories over the years of individuals not having estate planning. I even had personal experience with an instance where a decedent collected a whole bunch of fancy, italicized Latin phrases while auditing a college course and threw them into a handwritten Will. The court found this to be invalid and left the decedent intestate.

"Intestate" means that someone has died without a properly executed Will. In this case, the courts get involved with appointing someone to handle the affairs of the deceased.

I certainly was not going to become fodder for those stories while looking for a way to unload a bunch of owl-shaped knickknackery.

We celebrated my birthday (my natural new year) by going to lunch at an all-you-can-eat buffet that specializes in Mongolian cuisine.

I don't think I've ever put the words "Mongolian" and "cuisine" together like that.

It was awesome to hear the 1974 classic "Kung Fu Fighting" on the speakers overhead as I was ladling 'Kung POW' sauce onto my noodle and chicken concoction. That was right before my lunch was thrown on a hot grill by a non-Mongolian.

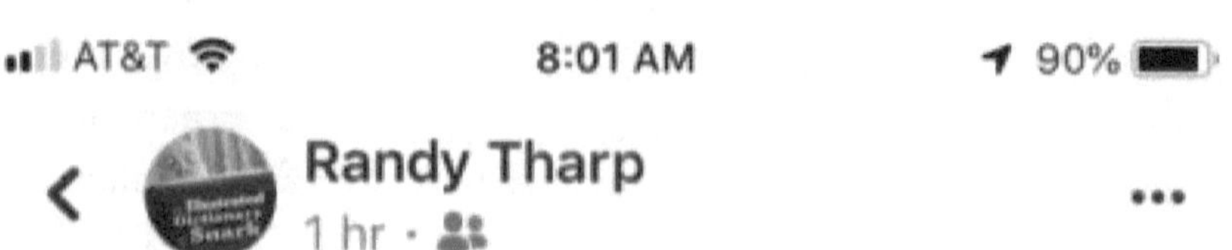

Later that day when we were back at apartment H, Mom approached me with a gift-wrapped box.

It should be noted here that three of my favorite things on God's Green Earth arrived on the scene in a five-year frame which occurred between 1977 and 1982.

It makes sense.

I ran across an assertion in a book about big data recently that most people (men more than women) pick their favorite sports team based on who was winning big at the time the burgeoning sports fan was approximately 8 years old.

That applied to me with football. I used to be a big fan of the team that lost the Super Bowl when I was eight.

The only reason I don't follow them anymore is because I don't follow the NFL anymore.

Going a little further on that one, I absolutely hate the team that won the Super Bowl that year I was eight and still do all these years later.

I would reveal what team that is, however, I won't for a couple of reasons.

Firstly, I never allow that team to be named in anything I write. To do so would lend credence to their cause and give them a platform I don't have to or want to give them.

The other reason stems from the fact that I've already alluded (or eluded, take your pick) to the identity of that team in a previous chapter.

Now certainly you may ask I why endeavor to burn so many calories on the hatred of a franchise within a league that I no longer follow.

My response is simple.

You don't have to follow the NFL to down vote one of their teams. I'm quite sure that's in the Magna Carta.

My favorite movie hit the theaters at that time as well.

A few years later, a comic strip appeared in the newspaper which rounded out the trifecta of the pop culture that would participate in the navigation of my life.

That strip was Bloom County by Berke Breathed. Over the years, I've collected books, posters, stuffed animals, and t-shirts featuring characters from that strip.

That should come as no surprise either.

Grandma collected cats.

Mom collected owls.

On a smaller scale, I collect selected pieces from the merchandising arm of the Breathed empire.

When Mom approached me on my 51st birthday with a gift-wrapped box, I groaned. Mom and I had agreed years ago that we weren't going to exchange gifts for birthdays, yet here she was making me feel like a jerk for receiving a birthday gift and not being prepared to reciprocate.

Granted the gift wrap was interesting enough to get my attention, because it featured Bloom County characters.

Okay Mom is off the hook a little for producing cool wrapping paper, but still on the fecal roster for getting me a gift.

With trepidation, I opened the box to find bubble wrap. I would need to set that aside for later.

All things being equal, I was around 8 or 9 years old when I discovered the dopamine hit generated by sitting there and popping bubble wrap.

It's not like I go out and buy bubble wrap just to pop it. At the same time, if I encounter some, I'm not going to pass up a wonderful opportunity to get a fix.

As I pulled out the first sheet of bubble wrap and set it aside for later, I found...

More bubble-wrap.

Mom must have remembered that I would appreciate the bubble wrap and put extra sheets in there. The alternative was that the gift itself was so fragile (must be Italian) that it needed some extra protection.

As I dug through the box, I pulled out sheet after sheet of bubble wrap.

Pop. Pop-pop. Pop.

And then, the box was empty.

"Happy Birthday!"

Nice.

Mom had just gotten one over on me by giving me bubble wrap in a box wrapped in Bloom County wrapping paper.

Best 51st birthday ever.

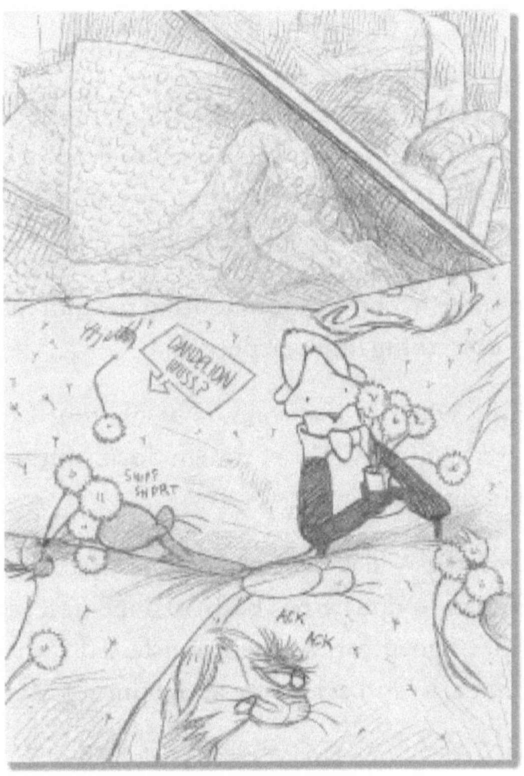

A few days later, on the morning of her 75th birthday, Mom and I packed up in her low-mileage, 2011 Subaru Outback and drove to an industrial park where her personal trainer had opened a gym. We were going to get a workout in before going to the lawyer to finalize her estate planning.

The trainer immediately put me to work on the stationary bike and then some exercises where I was climbing over invisible fences.

For the record, I don't even climb real fences. Climbing invisible ones in pursuit of a good leg workout comes off as ridiculous.

Mom had been talking this guy up to me for the last few years as really keeping her busy during these training sessions. It would be interesting to see Mom put in a good workout.

Granted, she spent a better part of the hour shooting the bull with the trainer instead of hopping invisible fences with one of her favorite sons. A few months ago when we were planning this visit, I expressed to her that I would need some time to shower after the workout before going to see the lawyer. She initially didn't understand why I wanted to shower between our appointments.

Watching her burn some major calories shooting the bull instead of straddling invisible fences put everything into perspective.

Later in the morning when at least one of us had our cardio in, we found ourselves at the lawyer's office. All the pertinent documents had been drawn up, and Mom just had to sign them.

There was a form with the Will (typed, not handwritten) and other documents which Mom had signed to donate her body to a medical school in Colorado. On top of that was a signed form which transferred ownership of a certain low-mileage, 2011 Subaru Outback to me at the time of Mom's passing.

"Gee thanks Mom. Guess where I'm going to park it?"

The next ten minutes were spent with Mom explaining to her lawyer how the person she was designating as her Attorney-in-Fact and eventual Executor once got her to park her Outback out back the Outback so that she could take a picture.

As the lawyer covered the highlights of the medical power of attorney document, a sentence came up. "I prefer to receive care in hospice rather than a hospital as the end of my life nears." This covered all the bases, but somehow, I never thought that scenario would arrive.

Mom turned her head and looked directly at me. She then gave that glare as if I were some lady talking crazy in the dining room at a nursing home.

"I want to be absolutely clear. No western medicine." Mom was no fan of western medicine.

"I completely understand."

Mom continued her glare.

*I don't think you do. I am **very** serious about this.*

—Yes Mom, I do understand.

I understand that you and I have differing views on life, the universe, and everything.

I understand that you believe I'm going to cast your wishes aside and put you in the care of western medicine.

I understand that to take care of you, I will seek out western medicine to do for you what I can't.

I understand that the nature of your ailment won't require aggressive intervention on the part of western medicine, because to be perfectly honest, the only treatment for what ails you is taking care of your daily needs and long-term care. There will be no needles, tubes, or IV bags. There will be no doctors constantly poking, probing, and prodding the remains of your dignity. There will be no surgical procedures. There will be a prescription to enhance your appetite. When the time comes, there will be morphine to help reduce anxiety.

I understand that it will be my job to advocate for you and your care while doing everything in my power to carry out your wishes, as long as they are in your best interest.

I understand that the donation of your body to western medicine will be considered a beautiful gift to science which will aid in the training and education of emergency doctors and technicians.

I understand that I'll be in the best position to take care of you when the time comes. I think you understand that too, otherwise we wouldn't be here.

Now I have a favor to ask.

In a little over three years, I'm going to show up at your door just before lunch on a Friday. I'm going to ask you to come back to Texas with me so that I can take care of you. I know you don't relish the thought of returning to Texas, but I'm asking you to set that aside and come with me.

Do you think you can do that for me?

Mom kept that look on her face that she always displayed when she was skeptical of my ability to tell the truth. I would like to think that after all these years, she knew that I had given up on telling lies and was more in the habit of practicing radical candor.

She then broke her glare. "Okay."

In Case I Croak

———

From: Barb Tharp

Sent: Saturday, December 21, 2019, 10:51 AM

To: 'Randy Tharp'

Subject: bills

I was just recording my January rent on my "bills" spreadsheet (the water is prorated, so it varies by month & I just got the bill), so I just highlighted a month's worth of bills to see if my SS would cover it. Yes, it does – almost exactly, and that includes things like my monthly payment to be listed on the EC/BC practitioners' map, etc. It's pretty much everything, but groceries & misc., but I didn't include the pension in the calculation, so that would easily cover groceries, and a few misc. purchases. So my practice is "gravy," but I really couldn't live without it, and Brandi says it's not an option as it covers her food, treats, and patches to keep her out of pain.

And BTW, not that I'm expecting anything to happen for a long time, but if it should, there's an Excel spreadsheet in documents on my computer, entitled THINGS TO KNOW IN CASE I CROAK. It explains my financial spreadsheet and other things and then lists various items (mostly some sort of décor) throughout the apartment, explaining sentimental value and also possible real value. That's the thing that's complete, but I was trying to get it somewhat in the order of what you'd see as you walk into the apartment, and that is nowhere near done. I just didn't want you to throw everything in the dumpster when you might be able to get some real money for some of it.

As I read thru the document, it already needs some updating, but I have higher priorities today.

———

From: Randy Tharp

Sent: Saturday, December 21, 2019, 10:55 A.M.

To: Barb Tharp

Subject: Re: bills

Understood.

Can we come up with a term other than "croak"?

Officially signed with the initials of one of the great grandsons of an outstandingly Prominent Citizen.

RGT

From: Barb Tharp

Sent: Saturday, December 21, 2019, 1:02 P.M.

To: 'Randy Tharp'

Subject: bills

I kinda like croak! What's wrong with it? The more reverent term that I use is transition. Will that work?

By the way, what's with that signature on your email?

From: Randy Tharp

Sent: Saturday, December 21, 2019, 1:30 P.M.

To: Barb Tharp

Subject: Re: bills

Yeah it's better than 'croak'.

The signature is a tip of the cap to your Grandfather.

He wrote a note to you back in 1964 when you were working as a librarian. He called you a "barbarian". After reading it a few times, I realized he was making a joke by combining your name and occupation.

The note was signed with a declaration that he was an "outstandingly Prominent Citizen". Naturally, I felt compelled to appropriate it.

Good ole Walt.

Officially signed with the initials of one of the great grandsons of an outstandingly Prominent Citizen.

RGT

From: Barb Tharp

Sent: Saturday, December 21, 2019, 1:45 P.M.

To: 'Randy Tharp'

Subject: bills

"Barbarian"? I don't remember that.

From: Randy Tharp

Sent: Saturday, December 21, 2019, 2:30 P.M.

To: Barb Tharp

Subject: Re: bills

Here's the text:

Georgetown, Texas, June 14, 1964

This is to certify that the undersigned has recently received a card from the public library at San Angelo, (formerly known as "Over the River") Texas. The same was typewritten but the inexperienced and inefficient typist failed to put periods after initials and at the ends of several names or titles. Am sorry they have to employ partially educated workers who, evidently, should bear names indicating that they are barbarians.

Officially signed with the initials of an outstandingly
Prominent Citizen.
W.E.S

Tharp 2.0 er... 4.0

The last time I composed a narrative about a multi-day event in which I was one of the chief players, the story played fast and loose with the events around the 1994 MLB All Star Game.

Remember that one?

That was the one where the players went on strike shortly afterward. There was no World Series that year.

I watched that game from a labor and delivery room. After the game was over, Wifey or someone else who was in charge announced it was time to get this kid born.

After lots of pushing, pulling, grunting, huffing, and puffing on the part of Wifey, the highly trained medical professionals who were working the room (and womb), and me, my son arrived at 5 a.m. the next morning.

Mom came to see us shortly after Junior's arrival. I have just a few memories of that visit. One was going out for Mexican food. I'm pretty sure Mom ordered chile rellenos. The other memory was seeing her off at the gate at the airport as she complimented Wifey with tears in her eyes. "You did a good job."

Within a few years, we welcomed a second-hand computer complete with word processing capabilities into our loving home. The first thing I did with that glorified paperweight was to recount the days around the birth of my son. I printed up several copies on the dot matrix printer, which accompanied the paperweight and circulated it among friends and family. This was long before I had access to the internet or even my own website, so I never really did anything else with that story.

Twenty-eight years later—almost to the same July week—I loaded Mom into a low-mileage, 2011 Subaru Outback and pulled away from the downtown cantina, where brunch is chile rellenos served by a rainbow-scented waitress with brown eyes disguised in blue.

We were on the way to see that kid who ushered in the 1994 MLB players strike, my favorite daughter-in-law, and their newborn son.

A few months prior to his birth at a baby shower, an in-law had ascribed the name of 'Tharp 2.0' to the kid because his name had not been announced yet.

There was great consternation among the various in-laws when they learned that Wifey and I had known the kid's name for the last six months and kept it a secret.

If you count the generations of living Tharps in the immediate family tree, this kid would be 'Tharp 4.0'. 'Tharp 2.0' would be those of us Gen-Xers at the grandparent level.

Tharp 4.0 and his parents had recently moved in with his maternal grandparents, so Mom and I set course for the 'burbs in northern Dallas.

Navigation on a smart phone is a kinder and gentler nation to me when I'm not downtown in a city I dislike, and I'm headed outbound. Certainly going northbound in Dallas wasn't the fastest way to get Mom home, but it was part of the mission I started in April to put her in touch with her great grandson.

We were met on the driveway by Tharp 3.0, who promptly helped Mom out of the passenger seat of her low-mileage, 2011 Subaru Outback.

A few years ago, Tharp 3.0 had gone with a group of friends to Colorado Springs on a ski trip. Since Colorado gets more snow than Texas, it only made sense to approach a ski trip in that fashion. While they were there, Junior took the occasion to see Mom.

Prior to that, I had taken him and Juniorette to see Mom in 2009 to help get her settled into her new house. Aside from watching Junior absolutely pummel Juniorette in their first and only (to date) snowball fight, the most memorable event of that trip involved some faulty plumbing under Mom's kitchen sink.

The realtor she worked with had done some remodeling of the kitchen for her and did a poor job of attaching the P-trap under the sink. This resulted in some minor flooding and gave me the opportunity to enhance my own plumbing skills.

Granted the term "enhance" would have been generous at the time. The more apt term would have been "develop".

This was prior to the days when I would take to the internet to obtain all my weekend-warrior and home improvement skills. Instead, I got pointers from the grizzled old man in the orange apron working the plumbing aisle at my favorite hardware store (aka "The Toy Store").

Irregardlessly, we got the issue fixed and I thought we were done with it.

The next day, the realtor showed up to finish some work he had started in the kitchen. I mentioned in passing what happened the night before and let him know I got the matter fixed.

Moments later Mom appeared in a pair of light blue flannel pajamas adorned with cartoon moose in a variety of poses and activities.

She had the look on her face.

I knew that look.

It was like the "That lady is crazy" look, but it was fiercer.

"Morning Mom. Nice jammies." My pleasantry was ignored. One doesn't thank their 40-something year old son for a sarcastic compliment and chew out the source of a minor water disaster in the same breath.

No, you go right to berating the culprit without acknowledging the remark about your whimsical sleepwear.

At least that's what Mom did.

Later that day when the relationship between Mom and her realtor/home renovation novice had been irretrievably broken and I knew a little bit more about the plumbing under the kitchen sink, Mom took us to 'yonder hill' to see what all the excitement was about.

One of the cool things about Pikes Peak is that they have a cog train that takes people up the mountain. We couldn't go all the way up that day because there was still snow at the top covering the tracks.

Instead, we went up as far as we could, made a pit stop and then came back down.

On the way back down, I developed an earache.

A nasty one.

That wouldn't have been so bad if I weren't getting on a plane later that day. On approach to San Antonio, the pain was so unbearable, I was hitting the call button trying to get something to knock me out.

I guess I held myself together and didn't create a viral incident worthy of being posted to the web.

I was diagnosed with an ear infection a few hours later.

I always wondered if that infection had anything to do with the exposure to the moose jammies.

But I digress.

Tharp 3.0 went to see Mom in Colorado a few years ago and had a pretty good relationship with her.

As we arrived at their house in the 'burbs, we sat Mom down and put Tharp 4.0 in her arms.

Everything I had been working for with Mom since last April was now complete. I had gotten her to Texas so she could meet her great grandson.

All that other stuff would be dealt with later.

We stayed for a while and visited with the kid, his parents, and his other grandparents.

And then, it was time to embark on the final leg of the journey.

Just A Bum On The New York Streets

Chowsky was more than just the name appearing in my first email address and the URL on my first website..

Chowsky, or a modified version of that name, was more than inspiration for the password I would use to get into MySpace.

Chowsky was more than just the answer to a security question which could be used to unlock the digital wallets for my crypto-currency.

It should also be noted that Chowsky is no longer used in any of my passwords or other security questions. All of you social engineers will need to take another approach at cracking my non-existent crypto-wallet.

In 1978, Dad had a salesman working for him who had a fertile Malamute of the female varietal. At some point during the year, that Malamute made the acquaintance of what was assumed to be a fertile Chow with a male libido powerful enough to propel him over the fence.

The result of that chance encounter (puppies, in this case) gave the owner of the Malamute the opportunity to use persuasive tactics on his boss. After all, he was a salesman.

Those tactics were the same ones Mom and Dad had fallen for over a decade earlier, when Uncle Roy pawned off our first dog, Dodger—a Border Collie-Spaniel special edition, courtesy of one un-neutered male and one un-spayed female who proved their fertility beyond a shadow of a doubt.

Back then, science was easier to trust.

A few weeks before Christmas that year, Dad came home with the cutest little puppy that looked like a cross between a Chow and a Husky. Dad put those two together and came up with the name Chowsky.

Full grown, Chowsky was a big boy (fertile and un-neutered).

One of the pictures in that cube I grabbed from Mom's desk back in Colorado features Chowsky. The focus is on a plate of Mom's chocolate chip cookies sitting on the table. Thumper and I are standing in the background, holding Chowsky up to the table. The picture was taken to celebrate his birthday.

Two things come to mind.

Number one, let's talk about Mom's chocolate chip cookies.

I married the woman who could make chocolate chip cookies as good as Mom's. Granted, the woman I married would be offended by the mere suggestion that her chocolate chip cookies are "as good as" Mom's. Wifey would expect a more generous and accurate characterization about the quality of her chocolate chip cookies.

The other thing that comes to mind was the ongoing thought in the house back then that I may not live up to my full potential.

There were no behavioral issues or anything like that which could put me on a first name basis with the principal, the guidance counselor, or a beleaguered probation officer. Either I couldn't focus on what mattered, or I wouldn't focus on what mattered at the time.

Things got worserer a few years later when Mom and Dad divorced.

I'm just thankful I had those issues and resolved them before Big Pharma and Big Tech took over the world.

One night at dinner, while sitting at the same table where Chowsky was denied chocolate chip cookies for his birthday, Mom, Dad, Thumper, and I gathered for a helping of some gosh-awful meatloaf and a side of green beans. Over the course of our delightful dinner conversation where my lack of focus and effort was the subject at hand, Thumper chimed in with his own unsolicited and unappreciated observation about his older brother.

"Randy's going to grow up to be a bum on the New York streets."

That jab stuck with me for many, many, many years, and I absolutely hated it. Even to this day, Dad brings that one up on occasion when reminiscing about the old days.

On a side note, I don't know if it was Mom or Dad who came up with that meatloaf recipe . I expect the meatloaf that Wifey makes is much better, however I've never had it. No matter how fancy you dress it up, meatloaf is the unfortunate coupling of hamburger and ketchup thrown into a casserole dish. I'm a hard pass on such heresy.

Humans sometimes eat this thing called "meatloaf," and it's unclear to me why. It's ketchup mashed up with onions and processed cow meat that was deemed unfit for steaks or burgers. There may be good meatloaf somewhere in the multiverse, but I haven't found it yet.

Mann, Kyle; Berry, Joel. The Postmodern Pilgrim's Progress: An Allegorical Tale (p. 137). Salem Books. Kindle Edition.

The four of us who were at the table gagging down that cacophony of ground meat and tomato sauce achieved success in our lives over the next forty years. The success just came as we broke up that group.

The slapdash prophetic gauntlet that Thumper laid down over a nasty plate of meatloaf never came true. Certainly, I've wandered the streets of New York City, but never as a bum.

There was a point in my college and post drop-out years where I wondered what my calling in life was to be.

What if I couldn't find one?

Was Grandma going to swoop in and dictate that I pursue a career in journalism? After all, one of those kids she mentored back in the old days pursued journalism and was flourishing in his career at a newspaper in western Texas.

Furthermore, I had previously shown some dexterity with the written word, and maybe one of my early interests should be fed so that I could earn a buck on the New York City streets as a journalist whenever I was in respite from my career as a bum.

At some point during that first year we were married, Grandma pulled Wifey aside and outlined the future, "Randy is going to go back to school and finish his degree in journalism and get a respectable job where he can support you."

At the time, I was working in the call center for a 24-hour cable shopping network where hosts like Mike Rowe convinced viewers that it was okay to purchase cubic zirconium, Thomas Kinkade prints, karaoke machines, and other knickknackery on creative installment plans.

Grandma didn't really understand the concept of cable shopping and found the whole practice to be disreputable.

Mike Rowe, on the other hand, would go on to do many other things in the years following. He's hosted several TV shows, advertised vehicles and appliances, and has done plenty of voiceover work.

That's right, Mike Rowe and I worked for the same company thirty years ago.

But enough about my six degrees of separation with celebrity. Let's get back to Grandma directing my future.

Of course that was going to work.

After all, Grandma made a similar edict when it came time for Mom to select a course of study and eventual career. That worked like a charm.

In the sense that it didn't.

For the record, Mom never went out of her way to hang a framed degree in Library Sciences from North Texas State University on any of the cubicle walls that encapsulated her while she worked as an accountant. For that matter, I don't think I've ever seen that document. I'm guessing it's been filed away using a three-digit code and a decimal point that only Dewey could find.

I opted to take the solipsistic approach by pursuing opportunities which were consistent with my own lofty delusions of grandeur. That was irregardlessly on the alternative view Grandma held about who should drive my destiny.

Journalism wasn't even the type of writing I wanted to do.

Journalism is up there with brunching on meatloaf when it comes to practices to avoid.

I'm going to look back on the prospects of being a journalist and/or a bum on the New York streets as bullets well dodged.

Even still I didn't know my calling, I didn't know if I wanted to capitalize on writing.

Some people are called into the ministry.

Others are called to be the ace relief pitcher whose game-saving, split-fingered monkey ball will make plate-crowding batters consider whether they ever got right with God.

There are those who are called into politics so that they can join the tyranny.

Besides exercising malapropisms, using words that don't really exist, and ending sentences with the occasional preposition, what was I called into?

On the day I turned forty, I began work in my current role. I manage complicated events which have many moving parts. In the process I deal with colleagues from multiple departments who reside way below and way above my pay grade. I also deal with similar colleagues who work outside of the organization.

That makes me an air traffic controller for the mutual fund industry.

I can't say I really went to school to learn about the work I do now, but maybe I did.

I spent about six years bouncing in and out of college majoring in data processing, journalism, and business. One of those disciplines may have been encouraged by an outside party.

I may have picked up some of the foundational elements of my work during my school years, but my present employer wasn't resting on those laurels when they were flipping quarters on whether I would be a good fit as a participant of their generous retirement plan.

Instead, they were more interested in the customer service and phone experience I had gained fielding calls from people using creative installment plans to buy cubic zirconium, Thomas Kinkade prints, karaoke machines, and other knickknackery from a 24-hour cable shopping network.

I started out with my current employer fielding calls from shareholders and their financial advisors. I also processed a whole lot of the work they sent us. I worked for ten years building a foundation in the industry basics before I stepped into my current roll of directing traffic.

But was this my calling?

When Thumper the amateur guidance counselor suggested I was going to be a bum all those years ago, could I resist the urge of grabbing a handful of that gosh-awful meatloaf and jamming it in his face while directly asserting that I was going to manage complicated events in the mutual fund industry?

Twelve-year-old Randy didn't even know what a mutual fund was.

So what was I called into?

The answer came to me during those months leading up to the point when I flew to Colorado Springs to get Mom and bring her back to Texas either seated comfortably in the passenger seat or bound and gagged in the cargo hold of her low-mileage, 2011 Subaru Outback.

While discussing the issue with Thumper one night, he made the passing remark to treat the issue with Mom like a project.

*A project? I am **not** a project!*

Of course.

The issue with Mom would be a complicated event with many moving parts. I would have to deal with multiple people including Mom's billers and friends, our family, the hospital staff, the staff at Los Prados Verdes Center for Nursing & Rehabilitation, and even Mom herself.

My call was to help Mom with the end of her life, and I had unknowingly spent the last 35 years training for it.

Blue Rivers Hospice

Chaplain Joe

When I put Mom into hospice care, I developed the slow-moving epiphany that my days of visiting her at Los Prados Verdes Center for Nursing & Rehabilitation were coming to an end.

I didn't know if that was good or bad.

That person in room 209 whom I called Mom was a mere shadow of the woman I brought to Texas last year in her low-mileage, 2011 Subaru Outback. For that matter, the woman I brought with me was a shell of the woman who had put me in charge of her affairs and well-being four years ago on her birthday.

That woman was gone and had been for a while now.

What good was it for her to lie there in bed all day being fed applesauce and berry flavored protein drinks?

All the anticipation and waiting turned my anxiety up to eleven. I started to get that look from friends and family who knew what the situation was.

Mom and I were ready for her suffering to end.

My suffering needed to end.

I was ready for the questions from concerned loved ones to end.

The calls, texts, and cards from Mom's friends needed to end.

Managing her personal affairs needed to end.

People were leaving me alone because they knew I was busy with something more important. That needed to end.

It all needed to end so that my life could get back to...

Normal.

The problem was that something worserer had to happen before things could get better.

Worserer?

I didn't know how long it would take, but a movie line I had quoted for years as a pithy little space filler became more poignant.

"Hurry up and wait."

The problem was that I didn't know exactly how much to "hurry up".

Did I have all her affairs in order?

Who did I need to call when I got the call I didn't want to get?

Did I need to be by her side day and night until the time came?

All that went through my mind yesterday, the day I signed Mom up for hospice care.

Now, I was back in the office doing my best for the mutual fund industry while giving my personal anxieties a break.

Ooga-Chaka, Ooga-Ooga,

Ooga-Chaka, Ooga-Ooga,

Ooga-Chaka, Ooga-Ooga

"Hooked on a Feeling" is a 1968 pop song written by Mark James and originally performed by B.J. Thomas. Many years ago, I created a snippet of the opening chant from the 1974 version of that song performed by Blue Swede and made it my ring tone.

Once again, I had my earbuds in, so that chant didn't break the sound barrier within the aisle of cubicles where I was planted.

Here in the information age, I get way too many calls from people trying to convince me to purchase solar panels, vacation packages, and Medicare plans. Sometimes I take the calls just to mess with them, other times I take the calls to make them question their employer's insistence on violating the "Do Not Call" laws that do such a good job of keeping the unwanted calls flowing.

This call was different, though.

It wasn't from Prados Verdes like the day before when Bobbie called. The caller ID had a name attached.

Joe T.

"Hello?"

"Hi this is Chaplain Joe with Blue Rivers Hospice calling for Randy Tharp."

Uh-oh.

A member of the clergy, working for the hospice service was calling me. He had a calm and soothing voice designed to take the edge off.

I was getting the call I had been dreading.

Even worse, I was at the office.

"Speaking." I braced for impact.

"Oh hi Mr. Tharp. I'm just calling to let you know that I'm visiting with your Mom right now, and I'll be here daily while she's under our care."

Relief.

Naturally, I resorted to one of my bad habits of injecting humor into an awkward situation. "She's not giving you any attitude is she?"

I heard that.

"I'm sorry?"

"Oh I'm just kidding. I was afraid you were calling with other news."

Joe understood. We exchanged a few more pleasantries and then I answered some questions a Chaplain who works for a hospice service is bound to ask.

Over the following days, Chaplain Joe would call me just to check in and let me know that he was visiting with Mom.

Each time he would call, it would put me on edge. I developed that fear that I was getting something other than a check-in call.

There was one time he called, and it became obvious to me that the battery in his flip phone needed to be charged.

"Hi Mr. Tharp, it's Chap...

...about your...

Just a few..."

Uh-oh.

Chaplain Joe was experiencing spotty cell service and may have been telling me something beyond the fact that he was just checking in.

"I'm sorry Joe, you're cutting in and out. Can you repeat that please?"

"Oh I get bad... out here. I'll just... you."

And then the call dropped.

Uh-oh.

A few minutes later, a text arrived. "Hi it's Chaplain Joe. Sorry I get bad phone reception out here. I was just calling to let you know I was visiting with your Mom."

Text updates subsequently became the notification medium of choice.

Weekend At Barb's

One Saturday, as I was finishing my visit with Mom, we received a visitor in room 209 at Los Prados Verdes Center for Nursing & Rehabilitation. The last couple of days had been filled with a new roster of visitors and phone calls from the in-house hospice service.

In this case, the visitor was the weekend hospice nurse who was making daily rounds for all the residents who were in her care. As she opened the door, Mr. OK could be heard just down the hall, activating his customized call button.

"OKAAAY." It practically drowned out the music from the "Team Barb" playlist which was set up on the bedside table.

When hope was high

And life worth living

Bianca introduced herself and we exchanged the usual pleasantries while she checked Mom's vitals.

No song unsung

No wine untasted

She gave me a report on Mom's condition and then asked if I had any questions for her.

I didn't. I think I had asked all the questions I needed to ask to everyone who had contacted me in recent days about Mom's care.

"OKAAAY."

Bianca then made sure I had the 24/7 on-call service number and took her leave.

But the tigers come at night

And they turn your dreams to shame

"Okay, Mom, I'm going to get going. I'll be back tomorrow, though — okay?"

But there are dreams that cannot be

And there are storms we cannot weather

"OKAAAY."

Okay.

Mom looked at me as if there was something she wanted to say. I stood there for a moment longer to see if anything was forthcoming.

Randy, I'm tired of this.

When will it be over?

Have you noticed that I'm not even here anymore?

—*Yes Mom, I have. I haven't seen you in over a year. This absolutely sucks and I hate that this has happened to you. I know you had so many plans for the rest of your life and none of them involved being one thousand miles away from 'yonder hill'. I hate that I moved you all the way down here in hopes you could continue your life living with me, and then I had to move you here. My only hope now is God's Big Plan comes to fruition for you soon, so you don't have to go through this anymore.*

"Okay Mom. Good night. Love you."

Love you too.

I turned back to look at her as I left the room. Unlike other days, she was looking back.

I sure did hate leaving her there.

When will this ever end?

I was better once.

I was going to expand my business.

I was going to buy a house.

Now, I don't even know how I got here.

I don't know where I am. There are a lot of old people here. Nurses come into my room at all hours of the day either trying to feed me or changing my clothes.

That crazy lady delivers mail and the old man down the hall won't shut up.

"OKAAAY."

Randy tries to feed me. Sometimes it works, other times it doesn't. He just doesn't feed me the only thing I really want. I can't even remember what I want anymore.

Bobby comes to see me, and he brings a dog with him. He keeps showing me videos of dogs running around in the snow. He also changes the channel on the TV to watch sports.

Bobby does more to interact with me, and Randy just sits there in silence.

He gets that from me.

My arms hurt. My knees are bent all the time. I can barely move my head.

It sounds like Randy's talking to someone outside my door again: "Hey Martin, how are you?"

"Hey there's my buddy. It's good to see you!"

"OKAAAY."

"Likewise."

"Hey, I want to ask you something."

"Go ahead."

"You know Ellen?"

"Ellen, Ellen. Is she one of the nurses? I'd probably know her if I saw her."

"OKAAAY."

"No, she lived here."

"Oh, Ellen down the hall? She's a sweetheart."

"She passed away."

Silence.

"When did that happen?"

"A few weeks ago."

More silence.

"You know, Martin, I'm glad that she's gone Home. Honestly, I'm upset I couldn't think of who she was a minute ago and hadn't even noticed she was gone."

"How's your Mom doing? I'm hoping she pulls through."

"We're continuing to pray for her."

I had a dream my life would be

So much different from this hell I'm living

So different now from what it seemed

Now life has killed

The dream I dreamed.

<u>Sad Last Days</u>

Many years ago I posted a status update on one of my social media feeds pondering the tabloid headlines which speak to the sad last days of celebrities. I had been at the grock when I posted that update, and I couldn't get over just how many of those trash rags litter the racks in the checkout lanes.

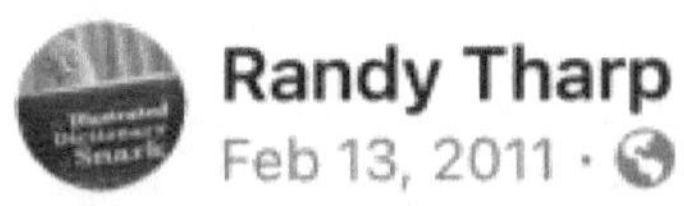

For the uninitiated, "grock" is the term Mom used on occasion when referring to the grocery store. Had "groshery" been spelled like it sounded, the term 'grock' would never have come into existence.

Granted, it wasn't as dazzling as when her father salted his lectures about Shakespeare's commoners with the word "irregardlessly", nor was it as baffling as when I toss around the word "worserer".

Irregardlessly, the word "grock" is challenging enough to the spellcheck algorithm within my own little digital Selectric. A quick adjustment to my customized dictionary will make things no worserer for the wear.

Back to a more blatant abuse of the Englitch language, I find the use of terms like "sad last days" on the covers of those rags to be gross and disgusting. That's irregardlessly of the fact that I find those rags and society's desire to keep up with the lives of said celebrities to be just as gross and disgusting.

The first time I ever encountered sad last days was in those months leading up to Dodger's passing.

That poor dog was tired and battling a few health problems. He was ready to say good-bye.

Mom suggested at one point that we may have to put him to sleep. Thumper and I got pretty upset about that suggestion. We didn't understand that letting the old man go would help to end some of the suffering he was enduring.

Looking back I wonder why Mom and Dad didn't make that decision. Maybe a consultation with the vet led them to believe it wasn't quite time to consider that.

After all, Wifey and I had a similar conversation with the vet about Faith six weeks before she passed.

Irregardlessly, Dodger was in his sad last days, and Thumper and I didn't fully understand what was coming.

When it came, it hit us hard.

It happened in the later years of our pre-teens when Thumper and I would spend the better part of our summer evenings hanging around the ballpark.

Thumper was in his last year of baseball as a 12-year-old. As for me, I had stopped playing a few years prior in pursuit of competitive swimming.

Dad was involved in the baseball league and served on the board of directors. He would be at the ballpark six nights a week during the season. Throughout the summer months, Mom would drop Thumper and me at the ballpark after she got off work. We would stay there for several hours watching games, horsing around in the wooded area behind centerfield, and playing pick-up games of cup-ball. At the end of the night, we would pile into Dad's medium mileage, 1980 Monte Carlo (company car) and head home.

Cup-ball was a lot like kickball.

The ball was a cup which had been reclaimed from the trash and subsequently wadded up into a ball-like object. It was then thrown by the pitcher (usually the kid who procured the cup) at the batter. The bat, of course, was the open palm of the batter. The ball-like object would be hit with the open palm of the batter with every bit of strength the kid could muster.

Once the ball-like object was hit and put into play, the batter would then become the runner on a shortened base-path which was defined by a light post, a discarded hot dog wrapper, and the nearest wood-paneled station wagon. Said vehicle was usually in direct line to field an errant foul ball from the baseball game being played on the adjacent field.

Outs were not defined in the traditional sense. Instead, the fielded ball-like object was thrown with great velocity at the runner. If the ball-like object hit the runner before the runner got to base, they were out.

In addition, there was a chance the runner would have a welt from the impact of the ball-like object. On top of that, a little bit of the pop (we didn't have soda in Wyoming back then) which had not been adequately emptied from the cup before it became the ball-like object would adorn the runner's Toughskins.

One late afternoon in August, Thumper and I were waiting for Mom to get home from work so that we could go to the ballpark. On these nights, we needed to feed Dodger and Chowsky and get them outside before we left the house.

On that day, Dodger had been in the basement with us. The challenge was getting him to go upstairs so that we could put him outside.

He didn't want to get up, so Thumper and I resorted to actions we had only seen Dad successfully pull off.

That's right.

Thumper and I picked Dodger up and carried him upstairs.

Every time we previously tried to pick him up, he would snarl with disapproval. After all, Dodger was the bull-goose loony and was not going to be carried around by a couple of boys who had less tenure than him.

This day was different, and we were able to get him upstairs and out to the backyard.

We put food into dishes for both Dodger and Chowsky and then adjourned to the ballpark.

We had only been at the ballpark for an hour or two, carrying out our standard agenda. Thumper was off playing cup-ball or something, and I was watching a game when I heard Dad call out to me from the league office. "Randy, get Bobby. We need to go."

"But we just got here."

"Get Bobby and let's go."

Dad didn't really have to tell us what was going on once we packed into his medium mileage, 1980 Monte Carlo (company car).

Dodger had died that afternoon out in the backyard when no one was home. Mom arrived home first to find him by the back porch and had put a towel over him.

When Dad, Thumper, and I got home, Dad proceeded to dig a hole near the back fence. Thumper and I stood there watching as we wailed and blubbered. It wasn't very becoming of a set of 12 and 14-year-old boys to carry on like that.

The next morning, Thumper and I woke up late in the summer morning like we normally did. Both Mom and Dad worked, so we were there by ourselves to cause whatever trouble came to mind.

This morning was different because we were still mourning the loss of one of our dogs.

A familiar noise emanated from the kitchen area which was attached to the garage. The noise was the garage door opener.

It wasn't necessarily the sound my phlegmatic washing machine makes when it's trying to spin my vast array of dark solids and plaid delicates. That, of course, is the sound of the opening chant inserted at the beginning of the 1974 Blue Swede remake of the 1968 pop song "Hooked on a Feeling" which was written by Mark James and originally performed by B.J. Thomas.

Instead, the garage door opener sounded like the underlying chant from the 1959 song "Running Bear" by Johnny Preston. As you may recall that chant is what inspired the chant at the beginning of the 1974 Blue Swede remake of the 1968 pop song "Hooked on a Feeling". That chant eventually became the standard ringtone on my phone many years later.

The garage door opener had been activated. The noise of that opener was accented by another familiar noise created by the diesel engine of Mom's medium mileage, 1981 Oldsmobile Delta 88.

For reasons unknown, Mom was not at work. She was pulling into the garage.

Thumper and I did a quick inventory to determine if Mom had come to take us somewhere we needed to be this morning.

After all, we were at that milestone in our lives where our teeth had been affixed with metallic bands and wires which were periodically adjusted by a sadistic Greek fellow who had advanced degrees in dentistry and orthodontia, and an office just across the street from the hospital. The premise of such activity was to forestall the possibility of having a crooked grill in our eventual adulthood. In all our grief over Dodger's passing, maybe we had forgotten we had an appointment that morning.

A quick check of the calendar confirmed that we didn't.

We weren't even dressed and ready to go anywhere that morning anyway.

The door between the garage and the kitchen opened and there was Mom.

Correction.

There was Mom, holding a puppy.

There's something to be said for getting a new dog the day after you lose one. Maybe it's right, maybe it's wrong, I don't know.

Irregardlessly, we now had a new dog in the form of a German Shepherd/Husky mix who was given the name Ginger. A picture of her graces the picture cube/pencil holder that Mom kept on her desk all the way up until I moved her to Texas.

Over forty years later, we were now in a different set of sad last days which didn't involve any of our dogs.

Mom was in hospice care.

Suffice it to say, we didn't know how long this was going to last.

The failure to thrive diagnosis from last August when she was in the hospital still resonated. Mom had done well at Los Prados Verdes Center for Nursing & Rehabilitation. Up until June, she was eating more than just what the mint green cows of Brenham, Texas produced.

Whenever she was out of bed and in her chair, she gave me a bit of resistance training whenever I took her outside and pushed her around the outer rim of the parking lot.

She may have been providing some logistical support to that group of freedom fighters and malcontents who resided at Prados Verdes with her. There were rumors that a rebellion was in the works, and Mom's vantage from room 209 down one of the main hallways would have allowed her to signal her geriatric comrades in arms on whether the jig was up.

By mid-June, Mom began eating less. That was even with the appetite enhancer on board.

During that second week of June, Mom entered those sad last days that I abhor reading about in the checkout aisle at the grock.

The pureed entrees which were previously delivered on a tray in the dining room just weeks before were replaced with a liquid diet of berry flavored protein drinks, bowls of broth, and cups of applesauce, all served next to the bed in room 209.

The sad last days and the associated decline presented themselves daily.

Here's the problem with watching someone in their sad last days.

Eventually the sad last days will become a sad last day.

You know it's coming, but you won't know when. Every day of those sad last days, you prepare yourself that maybe that day will be the sad last day.

You'll hope and pray that the sad last day comes soon because more than one sad last day amounts to too many sad last days.

Even worserer, you'll feel bad for hoping the sad last day comes soon.

And then you must start saying "Good-bye".

I started having deep, heartfelt conversations with Mom that I should have had with her years ago when I knew there would be two participants in the conversation.

I voiced some mistakes I had made over the years and shared what I was going to do to make them right.

I told her about the story I was writing about a guy who flew to Colorado once to save his Mom.

In all that time, I repeated the same promise to her, "Mom when this is all over, we're going to take you back to Colorado."

Thank you.

How Fast & Which Way

———

"You have ruined that car."

Mom had that glare.

I'm sure I'm not the only member of my generation which fielded a simple, two-word statement that conveyed punishment was imminent if behavior was not corrected immediately.

"That's 1."

When Mom said that she was giving one or both of us to the count of three to knock it off before corporal punishment would be delivered with an orange Hot Wheels track known as "The Orange Paddle".

Mom had honed her skills with the delivery of that statement in our formative years, so much so that she got to where she didn't even have to break the sound barrier with it.

Instead, she could deliver it with a glare.

It all started earlier in the day on a drive out in the country when all the idiot lights in the console lit up at once. The engine sputtered, and black smoke billowed from the exhaust. The car then broke down.

We were able to get the car towed to a mechanic, who triaged the issue and made a call to Mom advising that the motor failed because it had no engine oil in it.

She then shared the news with me.

"How did I ruin it?"

"You didn't check the oil level. You didn't get the oil changed. If you had, you would have noticed it was running low and gotten oil into it." Her glare intensified as I started to question whether she knew how to blink.

Looking back on that indiscretion, the charge made complete and total sense.

I was sixteen and driving my first car that was burning or leaking oil.

A whole bunch of it.

One part of that discussion which never took place was the fact that I didn't know I was supposed to be doing that stuff.

No one had told me the high mileage, 1974 Ford Mustang II was leaking and/or burning oil. Mom even had a mechanic check the car out before she bought it several months before. Word one to that effect was not uttered.

No one had shown me how to check the oil, or where the dipstick was or anything else about the mechanical upkeep of a car. I was a kid with his first car that didn't know better.

I just took the blame for ruining the car because at the time, I didn't realize that a few things weren't quite adding up.

It dawned on me years later that I probably wasn't the only guilty party in that event.

I wonder if it ever occurred to Mom.

Forty years later, we were getting back on the road and heading home in a low-mileage, 2011 Subaru Outback in which I had checked all the fluid levels the day before while negotiating whether I could get gas into it.

The drive between Dallas and home in San Antonio will vary between five and six hours.

That depends on at least three factors.

How fast are you going? Have you been on the road since yesterday morning in your beloved mother's low-mileage, 2011 Subaru Outback, trying to get her into an environment where you can take care of her as the symptoms of dementia become readily apparent? If so, you're putting everything your right foot has to offer into the gas pedal to hurry up and get done with it all.

Which way are you taking? There's a toll road that runs parallel to I-35 that allows you to put everything your right foot has to offer into the gas pedal of your mother's low-mileage, 2011 Subaru Outback without the chance of making acquaintance with the good people of the Texas Department of Public Safety who call attention to the fact that you're exceeding the speed limit by at least 30 miles per hour. Taking the toll road keeps you from driving through Austin and is well worth the charge.

How many times will you be stopping at Buc-ee's?

There are two of them on I-35 between Dallas and San Antonio, and Texas state law dictates that motorists stop there to use their clean and expansive restrooms, sample their smoked meats, and purchase at least one bag of Beaver Nuggets.

Please understand at this point, any description I could offer of this sugar loaded snack could not do it justice. Many times in the past year when Tharp 3.0 or Thumper were coming into town for a visit, I asked them to bring me a fresh bag of Beaver Nuggets. Each time, they declined to even stop. They had lame excuses like "The baby was asleep in the car, and we went non-stop.", or "I had Maggie (Thumper's dog) with me and went non-stop."

"Tell that to the judge." I would respond as I sought out a way to report them to the Texas DPS for their inconsiderate breach of motorist protocol.

Irregardlessly, Mom and I adhered to state law when both opportunities to make a stop presented themselves on the way home. The first time, we used their clean and expansive bathrooms in the way they were meant to be used. We then purchased a bag of Beaver Nuggets and a few drinks and got back on the road.

A little further south, we took the exit to the toll road, and we really opened 'er up in that low-mileage, 2011 Subaru Outback. No idiot lights on the instrument panel flickered. No black smoke billowed from the rear. The motor didn't sputter. No acquaintance was made with any of the fine men and women who work for the Texas Department of Public Safety.

About an hour later, we got off the toll road and back on the portion of I-35 which encourages herds of slow elk to occupy the left lanes at a velocity consistent with that of a school zone. All of that so we could make our last stop at the second Buc-ee's on our route. We gassed up since I knew where to place the needle-nose pliers, we used the clean and expansive restrooms, and we purchased a backup bag of Beaver Nuggets for use later.

Our destination was right at 50 miles away, and as all final legs of a long journey go, it felt like it took us a few hours to traverse it.

We pulled up to the house around midnight.

Wifey was outside waiting for us, as if she had been tracking our progress for the last few days using the wonders of cell phone technology.

For the record, she had been.

As I turned the key to turn off Mom's low-mileage, 2011 Subaru Outback, I looked over at her. "Welcome home, Mom. I'm really glad you came."

"I am too."

Ooga-Chaka

Tuesday - 6:58 p.m.

I opened my ongoing text conversation with Thumper where we discuss Mom, the latest music we're not listening to, and how much it hurts to pluck that 6-inch strand of hair growing on our respective ear lobes.

So...

If I should get the call in the middle of the night, do you to know immediately or should I wait until morning?

Virtual keyboards enable all sorts of [sic] behavior in my texting, from spelling errors to leaving out words altogether.

Let me know.

You don't have to call.

Don't pull a grandma!

Not going to pull a Ruth.

I will call you immediately and not wait until after the honeymoon.

Wednesday - 4:30 p.m.

Since the point where we had changed Mom's status to hospice care, I spent several hours each day just sitting in her room with her. There was a point where I could give her water or a protein drink through a straw. On a few occasions, Mom ate some applesauce for me as well.

But then that stopped, and she wouldn't even swallow the water I would slip into her mouth.

During the previous weekend I spent the better part of all daylight hours with her. When it came time to return to work next Monday, I arranged to work in the mornings and take afternoons off to go sit with her.

In that time, I prayed over her, and I read a few Psalms to her. Otherwise, I sat there and read, finishing book after book at a faster pace than I normally do.

When the shadows of this life have gone

Wifey and Junior (Tharp 3.0, father of Tharp 4.0) appeared late one afternoon. My son was in town for a convention downtown and took the chance to see his Grandma Barb again.

The last time he was here was right before her birthday in early June. He had his wife and Tharp 4.0 with him back then. Mom was still alert at the time and was able to understand she had a visitor.

Like a bird from prison bars has flown

After the three of us visited with Mom for a while and talked to a couple of the nurses, we decided to leave.

"Okay, Mom we're going to take off. I'll be back tomorrow. Love you."

To a land where joy shall never end

I'll fly away

Love you too.

Wednesday - 11:16 p.m.

Ooga-Chaka, Ooga-Ooga,

Ooga-Chaka, Ooga-Ooga,

Ooga-Chaka, Ooga-Ooga

"Hooked on a Feeling" is a 1968 pop song written by Mark James and originally performed by B.J. Thomas. I had learned that just recently, and just realized that song is as old as I am.

I was asleep when a phone call triggered the opening chant from Blue Swede's 1974 version of that song. I sat up immediately and tried to navigate the sudden jolt into consciousness where just moments before I was dreaming about...

I don't remember what I was dreaming about.

All I knew right then was that I didn't want to be hooked on the feeling I was experiencing.

My heart pounded from being pulled from my slumber so suddenly. A name appeared on the caller ID I didn't recognize. I knew what this call was.

"Hello?"

"Mr. Tharp?"

"Yeah."

"Sir, I regret to inform you..."

<u>Wednesday - 11:23 p.m.</u>

The last time I had talked to Thumper on the phone, it was a year and a few days ago. I was driving a low-mileage, 2011 Subaru Outback with Mom in the passenger seat sometime around midnight deep in the skeevy underbelly of Dallas.

Just so we're clear, I'm of the belief that Dallas is a skeevy underbelly, so to be smack dab in the middle of it with precious cargo in tow, I was on edge.

I was looking for the right turn to get to Thumper's apartment. He was out there somewhere trying to flag me down without being incorporated into the windshield of a low-mileage, 2011 Subaru Outback.

I was frustrated and taking it out on him.

All communication I had with Thumper over the last year had been via text or face to face. We both knew that if I initiated a phone call, it was **the** phone call.

Seven minutes after receiving the call from the hospice nurse, I called Thumper.

I didn't wait for him to come into town for a visit so I could tell him face to face.

I didn't avoid ruining his late Wednesday evening plans.

Instead, I made the call.

A Year Ago, on a Friday Afternoon

"Look Mom, I am worried sick about you.

I haven't had a good night's sleep since April. As your emergency contact, I've gotten three or four calls in the last month alone from people I've never heard of reporting their concerns about you. I'm afraid that it's going to get worserer now that Brandi is gone."

Worserer?

Throughout it all, I struggled to maintain my composure.

"Your lease is up here at the apartment, and you haven't taken on any clients lately. I know you have all your friends and community here and you love Colorado. At the same time, I just can't handle the fact that you're here all by yourself in the state that you're in."

Mom sat there taking it all in.

"We've got a room all set up for you and a couple of dogs that will love you as well. I'm asking you to come back to San Antonio and live with us."

And then I shut up.

I've learned over the years that when you've entered a negotiation, you state what you want, and then you shut up.

If the silence gets awkward, embrace it and don't give in.

Put the ball in the other person's court, because if you speak up after making your request/demand, you've ceded victory to your counterpart.

An eternity passed while I embraced the awkward pause, and we stared at each other.

Maybe this is something I need to do.

I'm not moving around very well, and I don't seem to have the wherewithal to get anything done anymore. Poor Brandi lay there on the floor for several days before Cheryl came over and helped me take care of her.

Why couldn't I take care of her when she passed away?

My phone keeps dying, so I can't call anyone. I don't even know who to call.

I'm so hungry, but nothing tastes good anymore.

I have some money from the sale of the house, but there's not much left. I keep dipping into it to make ends meet each month.

I'm on the brink of a mental collapse, a physical breakdown, and financial ruin.

I've been trying to think of a way to ask you or Rob for help.

Unfortunately, it's not going to be as easy as me just moving in with you and resuming life as you know it.

I'm a different person now.

Even though you're getting here just in time, it's still going to take you until September to get this situation under control.

Before the summer is over, I'm going to lose the ability to communicate verbally with you in any meaningful way.

The next several months following that will be tough in figuring out how to pay for my care.

It's going to be next spring before you see some relief and things start running like clockwork.

By then, you'll feel better about the decisions you've made, right as they were, wrong as they felt.

Managing me is going to test your fortitude and your relationships, and I'm sorry for that.

When you come to see me in Room 209, I will glare often and it will devastate you.

That will be dementia.

I regret that it has to be this way with my mind failing a year before my body does.

I regret that I won't be able to express all of this to you in the way I want to.

I know that a lot of what happens in the next year will inspire you to write it all down for your blog or even something bigger. I regret that I won't get a chance to read it.

Thank you for doing this.

Do what you need to do and bring me back to Colorado when it's all over.

Mom finally broke the silence. "I've been thinking about returning to Texas."

I pulled out my phone and found the group chat I had with Wifey and Thumper. I then typed a quick message.

"She's in."

One Last Visit

I may have gotten back to sleep last night.

After talking to Thumper, my mind raced with all the things I needed to do.

Just breathe and take some time to grieve.

I'll always be with you. It's better to be with you this way instead of the way it was a few hours ago.

All the decisions which needed to be made have already been made. Don't worry about managing anything right now.

Just breathe.

I had to breathe.

It wasn't even midnight yet, and I was already on my computer creating a checklist in my 'Team Barb' folder.

At the same time, I couldn't quite go back to bed yet. I couldn't just tell the business analyst in me to chill for a moment while I processed what had just happened.

The business analyst took over.

I drafted a post for Facebook.

I drafted an obituary where I mentioned "yonder hill", mint chocolate chip ice cream, owls, and all of Mom's dogs ranging from Dodger to Brandi.

It was close to 3 a.m. before I was able to lay back down and close my eyes.

A few hours later I woke up and assured myself that the events of not only the last six hours, but also the last twelve months had not been a dream.

They were real, and Mom was gone.

"I'm just ready for all of this to be over." I had uttered those words to my wife just a few days prior when Mom's condition was getting worserer.

In my work life in the cubicle, there are still checklist items to execute once the big event has taken place.

We verify that everything behaved as expected.

We identify and clean up any fallout that occurred because of the big event.

We notify both internal and external parties of the big event.

When all is said and done, we conduct a Lessons Learned meeting where we call out what went well, what challenges we had, and what changes we should make for future events.

We create a document which outlines everything we did before, during, and after the event.

As I worked through my checklist that morning, I made some phone calls I didn't want to make and sent some emails, text messages, and other messages that I didn't want to send.

I completed the 'Notifications' section of my checklist and read the next item.

"Clean out Mom's room and talk to Martin."

Geez I usually try to do the hard stuff first to get it over with.

Martin wasn't only an interested party in all of this. He was emotionally invested.

Martin had spent the better part of his life in some sort of assisted living. He had sisters who were visiting him regularly. Otherwise, I can't even begin to count the number of neighbors he's lost over that time, or the loved ones of those neighbors who got to know him and then stopped coming around.

And I was about to add to that tally.

On many an occasion, he would be camped out in the hall outside of his room and would see me either coming in or leaving Mom's room.

"Hey there's my buddy. It's good to see you!'

We would exchange pleasantries and then he would ask about Mom.

"Well we're just waiting for the next step in God's Big Plan to take place."

Martin knew Mom was in an end-of-life scenario.

For the last month I had wanted to have that difficult discussion with him about how my daily visits were coming to an end. I just didn't know how to approach that subject with him.

Martin continued to show optimism for Mom.

"I'm hoping she pulls through."

"Thank you Martin, I appreciate that." Now I was going to have to have that discussion with him and say "goodbye".

As I pulled into the parking lot that Thursday morning and parked Mom's low-mileage, 2011 Subaru Outback in the same spot I always did, my heart pounded. I was nervous and I had a dry throat. Mom had left this place less than twelve hours ago, never to come back. This would be my last time there as well.

I opened the cargo door where I had suggested I may have to store Mom during last year's road trip. I had put a storage bin in there a few weeks ago in preparation for this exact occasion. All the framed pictures, the stuffed animals, and her clothing would be packed into that bin.

I didn't stop at the front desk to sign in like guests are encouraged to do or confirm that I was there to see Barbara Tharp. I didn't print up and affix a name tag sticker to my chest. I walked by the receptionist who was talking to someone else and headed straight for room 209.

Martin was dozing in his chair right outside of his own room across the hall. I always wonder about the sanity behind waking up residents of nursing homes, so I decided to pack Mom's room first.

One of the nurses on that wing approached me. I may have seen her before, but I didn't really know her. It was rare for me to be there on a weekday morning during her shift.

"I'm so sorry to hear about your mother. I had been checking in on her on a regular basis for these last few weeks."

"Thank you, I appreciate that." I grabbed the wreath off the door to room 209 and put it and the storage bin on the bed where...

"You know, we lost three people yesterday. One of them had been with us since right after we opened." I wondered if Linda, the President of the Residents was consulting a little black book filled with names and anticipated dates of matriculation. I wondered whether Prados Verdes had ever lost that many residents in a single day.

"Three? Wow you must have been busy."

We exchanged a few more pleasantries, and then I spent the next ten minutes packing up Mom's things. All the packing from last year's three return trips to Apartment H at Enchanted Springs in Colorado Springs—and all the miles in the air and on the road—led to a brief stop at room 209 in the Los Prados Verdes Center for Nursing & Rehabilitation, where I filled a storage bin with Mom's remaining belongings.

I packed up the pictures and assorted knickknackery.

I took her sunglasses and a box of straws out of the cupboard.

I went through the closet and packed her clothes, save for one dress.

That dress found its way into Mom's room and onto her body throughout her stay here. I had no idea where it came from, but I knew it never belonged to Mom.

For that matter, it didn't belong in room 209.

It didn't belong on this property.

It didn't belong in this universe.

It didn't belong on this timeline.

I've had this theory for years that there is only one fruitcake in the world, and it's just been re-gifted from one person to another every Christmas.

That dress was the embodiment of my "one fruitcake" theory. It was going to stay here.

Packing her things up was hard, but the harder part was next.

Martin was still asleep across the hall in front of his room when I approached him.

"Martin?" My voice was low and a little shaky. No response. "Martin?" Still no response.

A member of the housekeeping staff approached Martin and spoke to him in Spanish in a commanding voice. She needed him to move away from his doorway so she could clean his room. He nodded and wheeled himself out into the open hallway before realizing that I was there.

Once he made eye contact with me his face lit up. He put his hand out to shake mine and I took it. "Hey buddy, it's good to see you!"

I looked back at Mom's door where I had just removed the wreath minutes before. I still had his hand in mine in a perpetual handshake.

"Mom passed away last night." I could feel the tears welling up in my eyes and my voice was shaking. I was doing everything I could to hold my composure.

A flash of pain ran across his face. He put out his other arm to offer a hug. I bent down to receive it. Martin repeated the same speech he had been giving me every day for the last six months about coming to see Mom regularly because you never know what's going to happen.

"Yeah, I know. Even though we knew this was going to happen, it still hurts a lot." Any semblance of stoicism I was trying to display was packed up in the storage bin at my feet. "Tell you what, Martin. From that first time I came here back in September until now, it's always been a pleasure to talk with you. Whether you're aware of it or not, you've always made these visits easier, and I'll never forget that. I want to thank you for all of your support over this last year."

Martin nodded, still visibly upset.

"Okay I got to go now. You take care of yourself, ok?"

"Okay."

I was halfway down the hall which Mom would monitor for the benefit of the forthcoming rebellion the residents were planning when I encountered Nurse Bobbie. Just one short month ago, Bobbie had contacted me suggesting that hospice care may be a good decision. Bobbie expressed her condolences, and I thanked her for all that she had done for us in the last year.

As I loaded the storage bin into the cargo-hold of Mom's low-mileage, 2011 Subaru Outback, it occurred to me that I would never come back to Los Prados Verdes Center for Nursing & Rehabilitation.

My office was just a mile away, and I would never turn right out of the parking lot to get here again. Instead, I would turn left to go home.

Standing there in the parking lot at the back of Mom's low-mileage, 2011 Subaru Outback, I was reminded of a time I parked in that spot just four months ago.

Having lived in this region for well over 30 years, I've come to the conclusion that the best time to be here is in March and April.

The Texas version of winter (a sorry excuse for one for that matter) has left and now the Chamber of Commerce season has arrived in its rightful place ahead of consecutive days of triple digit heat moistened with just enough humidity to...

Metaphor and simile fail me right now.

I pulled into the parking lot at Los Prados Verdes Center for Nursing & Rehabilitation on a beautiful day at the end of March around 4:30 p.m. I parked in the same spot I always do because I'm a regimented creature of habit.

If Mom were up and at 'em, I would take her for a walk around the parking lot before wheeling her to the dining room for whatever pureed cacophony and other aural delights being served up for dinner.

After signing in, I made my way down the main hallway toward room 209 and saw that the door was closed.

This was a good thing.

This meant that a C.N.A. was in there getting Mom out of bed and dressed for dinner. This meant we could go outside for a walk instead of sitting around in her room watching the sappy movie *du jour* while waiting for the 5:00 p.m. dinner bell.

I waited at the 'T' shaped intersection which converged at room 209.

Just to my right, I could hear a discussion going on in Martin's room. It was Martin's birthday, and a few of his sisters had shown up to celebrate and decorate his wheelchair.

Martin had mentioned his upcoming birthday to me daily for the last few weeks.

Moments later, the three of them emerged. Martin's chair was decked out with all the subtlety that LED lighting and Mylar balloons had to offer.

"Hey there's my buddy. It's good to see you!"

"Good to see you too Martin. Happy Birthday."

"Thank you. How's your Mom doing?"

"Oh she's doing fine. They're getting her ready right now and then I'm going to take her outside."

"I was out there earlier. It's nice." Martin and his sisters proceeded down the hallway to take in more revelry that could only be delivered to the facility mascot.

At that point Ludy opened the door to room 209 to reveal Mom all dressed up and ready to go. I could always tell which C.N.A.'s were taking care of Mom based on her wardrobe and general appearance. There were some who did what they needed to do and that was it.

Get 'em outta bed.

Get 'em cleaned up.

Get 'em dressed.

Wheel them down to the nurses station to listen to stories from Doc Brown while waiting for their connecting flight to the dining room.

There were others who went beyond the call of duty.

They made sure that the resident wasn't only dressed, but they were dressed in matching colors.

That included socks and slippers.

They made sure the residents' hair was clean and combed.

Ludy was somewhere in between. She meant well, but just didn't seem to have a sense of finesse when it came to getting the residents ready.

Working with Ludy was always uncomfortable. Every time I encountered her, she would say the nicest things about me being the attentive son. The comments turned up the knobs on my imposter syndrome.

She meant well and generally disagreed with my harshest critic; me.

When the door to room 209 opened, there was Mom dressed in a seizure-inducing quantity and quality of colors. Her hair had not been combed, and a travel pillow had been affixed to the back side of her neck to keep her head from slumping to the side.

Mom just glared at me as I processed the results of Ludy's work.

Look at me!

I look ridiculous!

Where did I even get this ugly dress? Is it mine?"

—No I wouldn't have let you come to Texas with anything like that. I thought I was the only one who didn't like it. It must have been passed on to you before I could get some of your clothes over here.

"Get rid of it. It's hideous. I don't know why they keep putting this thing on me."

There were too many fire alarms around here to burn it. Maybe I could give it away by casually tossing it into someone's room when no one was looking.

A few minutes later we were at the front entrance of Los Prados Verdes Center for Nursing & Rehabilitation. Mom was now wearing the pair of sunglasses I kept in her room for such occasions. All the better to maintain her privacy from the tragic wardrobe choice her C.N.A.-of-the-day had made.

I made a left as we went outside. "Let's go counter-clockwise today." This would give me a slight rise at the back-end of the facility where the kitchen was located. It never hurts to get your flights in when you're building on the steps you've taken during the day.

We got to the back and there were no odors present that would reveal what was for dinner. We then took another left turn and traversed the back of the facility.

Oh look at that, you can see the cog train going up the side of the Peak. Do you remember when we took your kids up that thing?

—I sure do. That was the day you chewed out your realtor for doing a poor plumbing job on your kitchen sink. You were wearing those flannel moose jammies.

I also remember the nasty earache I got while we were on the cog train coming down yonder hill. It got worserer on the airplane on approach back into San Antonio that same day. I was in so much pain; I was ready to throw a tantrum on the plane and then be subdued by a Federal Air Marshall. I came out of all of that with a nice ear infection.

Um... For what it's worth, that's not the cog train going up the Peak, though.

No?

—No that's the roller coaster at the amusement park on the other side of the highway. Keep watching and you'll see that cog train plummet once it peaks.

Oh.

I thought it was the Peak.

—I guess it looks a little like it.

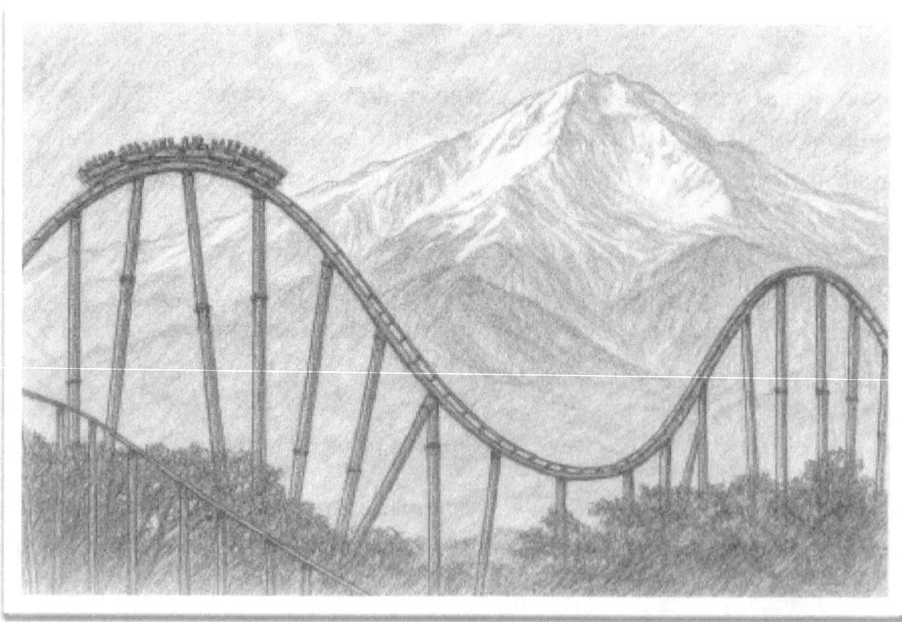

As we rounded turn three and made our way towards the front where most of the visitors were parked, I stopped at one particular car. It was always in the same spot when we took these walks.

"Does that car look familiar Mom?"

"Yes."

"What is it?"

"It's my Outback."

"Exactly."

"I'm wondering why the Outback isn't parked out back the Outback."

—Yeah, I guess I need to go do that.

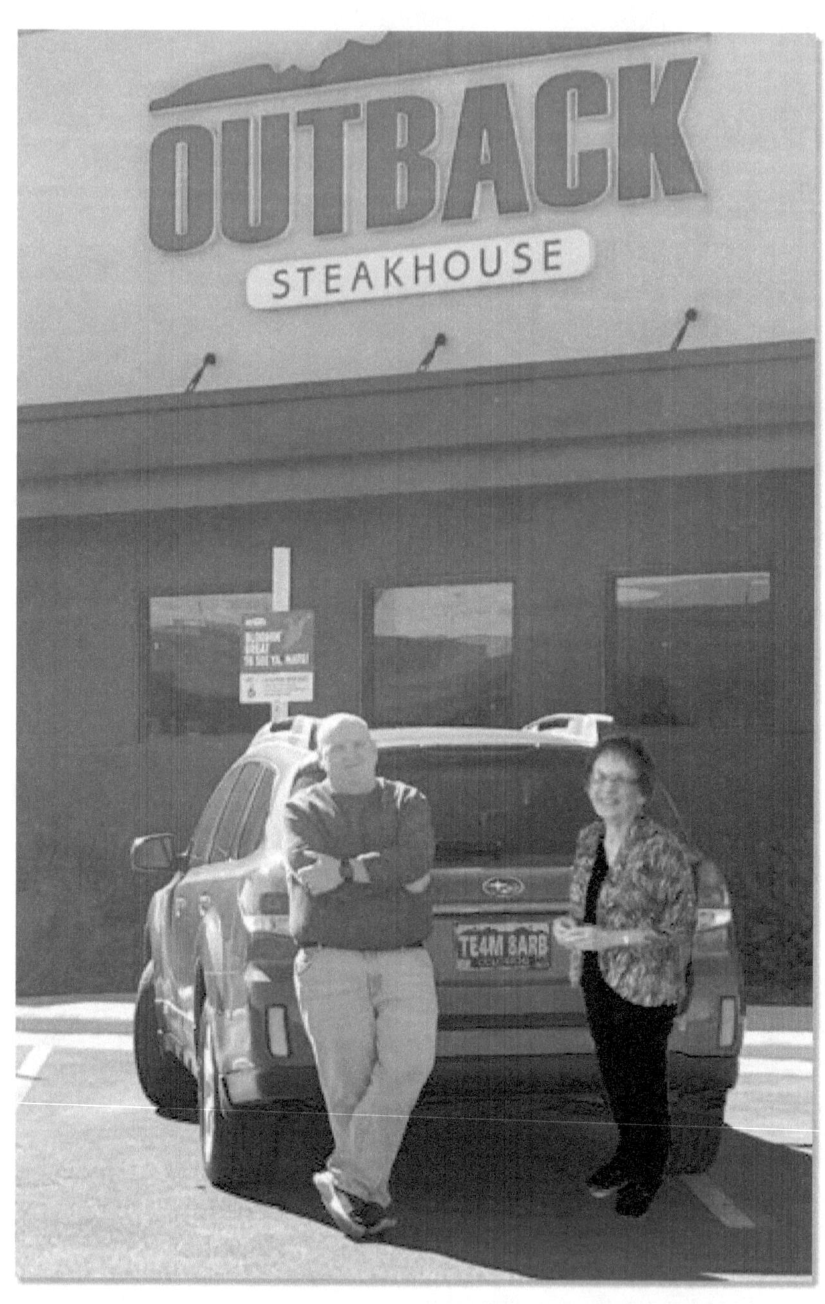

Randy and Barb, out back the Outback with an Outback

Afterward

As part of the estate planning Mom did four years ago, she filled out paperwork to donate her body to a medical school in Colorado.

Now that Mom was in Texas, giving her body to a school in Colorado wasn't going to be feasible. Making that last set of arrangements was the one thing I had been putting off with Mom's care.

By the time we put her into hospice care, it became a more pressing matter.

I was able to locate a service closer to home which could take care of Mom when the time came.

I had expected Mom would be with them for a year or two. Afterward, Thumper and I would take her back to Colorado.

A few months later, I got the following email:

From: J.L.

Sent: Thursday, October 5, 2023, 5:14:16 P.M.

To: Randy Tharp

Subject: USPS Delivery

Mr. Tharp,

Please keep an eye out for USPS to make a delivery of your mother's remains by 6 p.m. tomorrow (Friday, October 6th).

Sincerely,

JL, RN

Co-founder & COO

From: Randy Tharp

Sent: Thursday, October 5, 2023, 5:14:16 P.M.

To: J.L.

Subject: USPS Delivery

Thanks for the update J.L. I'll be on the lookout tomorrow.

Honestly, I'm a little confused. I was of the impression it would be a year or two before we got to this point.

Officially signed with the initials of one of the great grandsons of an outstandingly Prominent Citizen.

RGT

From: J.L.

Sent: Thursday, October 6, 2023, 8:55:06 A.M.

To: Randy Tharp

Subject: USPS Delivery

No sir, one year max.

Your mother was able to provide training and education to an amazing group of emergency medical doctors and technicians, as well as to a group that was compiling data for the FDA for a new surgical approach and closing technique.

Take care,

J.L., RN

Co-founder & COO

It's a bit ironic that as much disdain as Mom had for Western medicine, her last act was to help improve it.

Mom passed away a little less than three months ago, and I didn't expect to see her again for another year or two.

I wasn't ready to see her this soon.

Yesterday, our postal carrier found the doorbell button, which is conveniently hidden by some green growing thing Wifey has on a stand at the front door.

I was working from home at the time and on a conference call when the doorbell was activated. This prompted Charlie, our Silver Lab to let out an excited yelp advising us that someone was at the door. Under the assumption we didn't hear her yelp, she proceeded to the door and cursed the sad truth that she doesn't have the dexterity or opposable thumbs needed to open the front door. She left that task to me instead.

I opened the door to find our postal carrier with a solemn look on her face. The markings on the box she was delivering had abandoned all discretion about what was being shipped. It was marked on all sides that the contents were cremated remains.

Mom didn't arrive seated comfortably in the passenger seat or bound and gagged in the cargo hold of her low-mileage, 2011 Subaru Outback like she did a year ago.

Instead, she arrived courtesy of the U.S. Postal Service.

I wasn't ready for this.

The box sat at our table for a few hours before I got up the nerve to open it.

A note was placed at the top:

———————

———————————

I wasn't ready for this.

But then, things got a little better.

The box which was marked with the silhouette of an urn on all sides was about the same dimension as that box covered in Bloom County wrapping paper which Mom gave me four years ago for my birthday.

Same dimension, different weight.

Granted, there was just as much bubble wrap in that box with Mom as was in that box from Mom.

Pop. Pop-pop. Pop.

Acknowledgements

It's rare that when I finish reading the meaty and beefy guts of a book that I maintain full attention on the list of acknowledgements the author(s) make at the end. These are the people, places, and things (nouns mainly) who in one compensated or otherwise charitable way contributed to the verbal brilliance upon which I have just beset my slightly far-sighted, slightly astigmatic look-balls.

Even still, I feel compelled to at least skim the list so I can claim the bragging rights that I read that book from stem to stern.

Now, I find myself in a position to advise the reader the following material could be skimmed but would be better if read at regular speed so that it can trigger a memory or two about all the events (unexpected or otherwise) which took place in this narrative.

As with acknowledgements I've found in other books, I'll start with the standard phrase of "First and foremost".

First and foremost, Team Barb could not have been put into motion without the **grace** and **patience** of Beckie, my beloved wife of 30-sumthin' years. Throughout the whole 18-month ordeal, Beckie supported me the whole way. That first weekend I flew back to Colorado and left Beckie to take care of Mom nearly broke the both of them. Once we got Mom into the nursing home, Beckie was the one making sure that Mom had the types of clothing the C.N.A.'s suggested would be best. Something, something, stretchy-top. Beckie also included the entire staff at the nursing home as recipients of platters of Christmas cookies she makes every year. On top of that, she was making a wreath for each season to hang on the door of room 209.

I wish I could even begin to discuss the amount of **grace** and **patience** Beckie provided, but I just can't. Just understand that the fact those two words which garnered bold font treatment is the tip of the iceberg of what she gave at the early stage, throughout the middle, at the end, and even during the months afterward when I processed my grief at the computer writing about a low-mileage, 2011 Subaru Outback.

And then there's Robert, aka Thumper, my little brother of 50-sumthin' years. Rawb (as I call him) and I have a lot in common, but at the same time we're different. Most notably, I can tell when a brown-eyed girl is wearing blue contact lenses.

Rawb, not so much.

Irregardlessly (*there's that word again*), we have similar talent stacks born from our shared upbringing, and the careers we've pursued in what can generously be characterized as our adulthood. That allowed me to bounce any and everything off him to round out the approach to getting Mom to Texas where we could take care of her. Rawb was the first to signal that we needed to get Mom into a nursing home. Mom and I weren't quite ready to accept that yet.

When Rawb came to town to visit Mom he was pot-committed to spending every minute he could with her. That was opposed to just showing up at 'da home' (as he would call it), put in an appearance and then count down the minutes until it was time to leave. Those all-day visits that Rawb did that I could never do helped immensely and gave Beckie and I some respite to recharge. That's not to say that Rawb was nothing but a substitute. Rawb was Mom's other favorite son and just as dedicated and attentive to Mom's care as I was. He was there for Mom, and not for me. That's the way I wanted it.

Awesome parental support came from my Mother-in-Law Maxine Junek, and my father Ed Tharp. One thing I didn't touch on in this story is the fact that from that point in April when I had that troubling call with Mom, up until two days before I flew to Colorado in July to get her, I kept her condition a white knuckled secret from everyone but Beckie, my kids, and Rawb. My boss and a few colleagues knew the basics because I was about to disappear for a few days.

On the evening of my son's birthday, we had gone out to celebrate, and I pulled Maxine aside and told her what was going on, and what I was about to do. The first thing she did was offer the bed from her spare bedroom for us to set up for Mom. Beckie's **grace** and **patience** was impeccably sourced.

Later that night, I called Dad and let him know what was going on as well. Much like Maxine, Dad offered up all types of support, some of which I eventually accepted.

To my son Nick, his wife Valerie, and their son Isaiah, thank you for all your support. Nick helped to get the spare bedroom ready for Mom after I had already flown out. That visit to San Antonio and one of the missions I sent you on was a tough one, and I'm sorry you had to endure what happened back then. A few days later, Nick and Val along with her parents Frank and Barbara hosted Mom and me at their home in Dallas. It was there that Mom met Isaiah for first time. In the days leading up to Mom's passing, I was asked several times if Mom was holding on to see someone before she passes. I never really thought that was the case because everyone who could get there had visited and said good-bye to Mom. But then Nick showed up in town for a few days on business and came to see her. She passed later that evening.

I give a special thanks to my daughter Leighanne. That first month I had Mom here was tough because Lei was living here too. Throwing Lei into some of those situations was not fair and sometimes came out of an act of desperation on my part. There were many times I was an absolute jerk to her, and I regret that. Irregardlessly (Lei hates that word), we're in a better place now. I'd like to think she has some Iditarod Coins stashed in her purse.

During that first month when Mom lost her ability to walk, we were moving her around the house with an office chair. In stepped Beckie's brother Carl and his wife Bonnie with a wheelchair and bathroom chair. They had picked up this equipment for her ailing mother in the previous year. This helped immensely and we're forever grateful for their contribution.

There came a point where I needed to get some of the bigger items out of Mom's apartment. The plan was to fly up there during Labor Day weekend, rent a moving truck, and bring some stuff back. Rawb couldn't go, so I booked a flight for my son Nick to join me. A few weeks before the trip, Nick broke his leg on the basketball court against the pole holding the basket. I won't go into details about how that happened, save for the fact that Nick wasn't playing basketball at the time.

With Nick on the disabled list, I conscripted my nephew Max Swain to round out the brute squad that would accompany me to Colorado Springs. He then rode shotgun with me in a U-Haul that couldn't maintain adequate tire pressure on the rear passenger side. That happened all the way out of Colorado, through New Mexico, and onward to San Angelo where Dad lives. In addition to the house that he and his wife Marsha live in, Dad owns the house that Ruth bequeathed (via handwritten Will) to him in exchange for managing her estate all those years ago. Max and I stayed in that house that night before taking off the next morning, bound for San Antonio.

Some of the items that Mom had taken from that house when Grandma died came full circle to spend the night in the driveway thirty years later.

Thank you Max for all the help you provided. The things I saw you do to that Chicken 'n Waffle plate at the IHOP the morning we left Colorado Springs still resonates over a year later.

Thank you to Walter E. Suddarth for more than just a glimpse into my heritage on Mom's side of the family. I wanted so much to incorporate my great-grandfather into one of the scenes in the dining room but never found a good way to do it. His signature line alone is enough to inspire and aspire to be a self-proclaimed, outstandingly prominent citizen.

Thank you to his daughter Ruth, my Grandma. She was quite a character and left behind a lot of mixed feelings about some of the things that she did. I don't know, nor will I ever know, why she did those things outside of the fact they were within her psychological make-up.

Ruth did some interesting things in her time here. Most notable was a donation of a significant wad of cash to restore some stain glass windows at Oxford. I believe those were in the library where inexperienced and undereducated barbarians mistype names on library cards . That would have been right up her alley.

Let's not forget Prentiss (aka "Butch"), Ruth's husband, and my Grandpa. Without Mom's passing comment about him in the low-mileage, 2011 Subaru Outback on hot day in July somewhere on the southbound side of I-25, my insufferable use of the word "irregardlessly" in long run-on sentences would have come off as an undesirable and unacceptable assault on the Englitch language.

"Englitch?"

Let's talk about Los Prados Verdes Center for Nursing & Rehabilitation. I'm not going to reveal the name of the facility for a host of reasons. Most importantly, the staff along with the residents and their loved ones deserve their privacy. I changed only some of their names in this effort.

To Linda and Gwendolyn, thank you for making it a point to say "Hi" to both me and Mom at the same time. The consideration and hospitality you two showed through Mom's stay will not be forgotten.

To Ellen, I regret that I didn't realize you were gone until Martin told me. I think I was out of town at the time you passed. The fact I couldn't even think of you when Martin first mentioned your name still bothers me. Rest in Peace Sweetheart.

To Martin, what can I say that I didn't say that morning in the hallway? I meant every word of it.

To the entire staff at Los Prados Verdes Center for Nursing & Rehabilitation, I want to commend you on a job well done. It starts with the administrative staff who showed a great deal of patience with me as I worked through the financial aspect. At the front desk, there was Alex, Jacqui, and Bernadette who addressed me by name whenever I wandered in or out. At the back of the building there was the kitchen and dining room staff which made sure Mom had something decent to eat, even if she didn't want it. One member of that staff stands out to me as she always came over to say "Hi" and share pleasantries in her broken-Englitch. It turned out she was an engineer from Russia whose husband was here in the states. The custodial staff was good at keeping the entire facility clean and never gave me any cause for concern.

And then there was the nursing staff that drove it all home for me. The collection of Registered Nurses, Certified Nursing Assistants, and Medical Technicians provided the care for all of Mom's physical needs. They helped to preserve the dignity for Mom that Mom, Beckie, and I couldn't provide.

Just a few of their names come to mind right now, and several of them appear throughout the entire story. I wouldn't do any justice for the entire staff by calling out just a few.

The in-house Hospice service, whose company name I won't mention here because it would tie back Prados Verdes, was top notch as well. Everyone with that service who took care of Mom in that last month deserves my gratitude. That includes the Nurse Practitioners and Chaplain Joe who visited Mom daily.

Mom had friends checking in on her on a regular basis. First and foremost, there were the Sisters of Alliteration, Cheryl, Shirley, and Sheri. I don't believe these ladies have every met each other, but they all knew Mom. In addition, I would hear regularly from Mom's friends at the Center for Spiritual Living in Colorado Springs. All the cards, gifts, and well-wishes were always appreciated.

I want to thank everyone at work, both here at the office in San Antonio, and the other three offices in Virginia, Indiana, and California. The level of support I got from that whole group (too big to name them all) was outstanding.

But let's not forget the unsung heroes which have graced the pages in this narrative. These are the people, places, and things (more nouns) which contributed in their own way.

Firstly, whoever came up with the meme of "Out back the Outback in an Outback" needs a fist bump and a high five. I'm not sure I could have pulled this one off in my Ford Edge. I would have needed to abscond with U2 guitarist "The Edge" and the edge of a cliff to make that one happen.

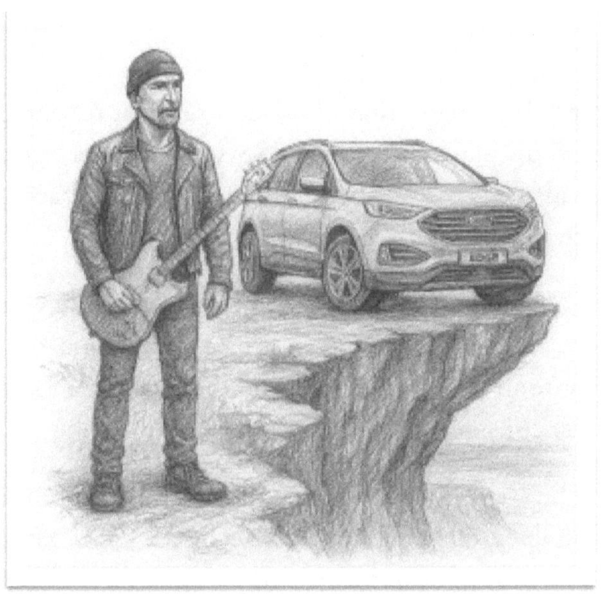

While we're on the subject, props to the good people at Subaru for giving us the Outback. In a related note, props also go to the inventor of the needle-nose pliers. Had it not been for a pair of those bad boys, I wouldn't have been able to get gas into Mom's low-mileage, 2011 Subaru Outback on the way to Texas.

I'd like to thank all the cows in Brenham, Texas who provide us with the base ingredient in Blue Bell Ice Cream. Mom loved your stuff.

Regarding vittles, I'll also send out gratitude to the Outback Steakhouse which provided a backdrop in the meme. Try the Tasmanian Chili. It's rather good, and it has no beans. Huhot is a close second. Mom introduced that one to us on a previous visit.

As far as travel is concerned, I'd like to thank the airlines I used to get back and forth between here and Colorado, but I can't. When I had to cancel Mom's initial flight to Texas to meet her great-grandson, they gave her flight credit that only she could use. That would have been fine if she were ever going to fly again, but she wasn't. A member of the escalation team tried to convince me that the extra travel miles they were giving Mom for the inconvenience was a good thing.

On the other hand, I do thank that nice lady I sat next to who perceived I was in a hurry to get off the plane. I also want to extend another heartfelt apology to that kid who got in the way of my surprise vomit cannon back in 1991. I hope that didn't have too many long-term effects on him.

Moose jammies! Watching Mom chew someone out while wearing those was a classic. A few years ago, I invested in a pair of sleeping britches that have silhouettes of moose all over them. Had it not been for that fateful day in 2009, I would have never considered them.

Thank you to all the artists who landed on the Team Barb playlist on my phone. Fleetwood Mac, Eagles, Glen Campbell, Creedence Clearwater Revival, REO Speedwagon, and a host of others provided a respite from the high-quality sap being broadcast on the TV at the time.

Christopher Lloyd gets a nod in all of this. Not only to inspire the Doc Brown character in the dining room (she did exist, and her hair looked like his when the right C.N.A. wasn't there to braid it), but also for giving me the idea that I could approach this story in a non-linear fashion.

Robert Kanigher and Carmine Infantino get some credit in all of this as the creators of The Flash. I don't know if they had any involvement in the story line of Flash engaging in time travel to save his mother. That story line has been run through the comics, an animated movie, the latest TV series, and the 2023 movie, so I've got to think it was part of the Barry Allen origin story at one point or another.

Dave Ramsey is a guy on the radio who helps people get right with managing their money. Had it not been for me to listen to his radio show, I wouldn't have pushed Mom to do estate planning all those years ago. I also wouldn't have sought out long term care insurance for her either. More importantly, my own financial house wouldn't have been able to run Team Barb in the way it needed to be run. Thank you for all the guidance Dave.

Finally, bubble wrap.

'Nuff said.

Soundtrack

Parton, Dolly. Lyrics to "9 to 5". RCA Nashville, 1980. Genius.com, https://genius.com/Dolly-parton-9-to-5-lyrics

Preston, Johnny. Lyrics to "Running Bear". Mercury, 1959. Genius.com, https://genius.com/Johnny-preston-running-bear-lyrics

James, Mark. Lyrics to "Hooked on a Feeling". EMI Svenska, 1974. Genius.com, https://genius.com/Blue-swede-hooked-on-a-feeling-lyrics

Owen, Randy. Lyrics to "Mountain Music". RCA Nashville, 1981. Genius.com, https://genius.com/Alabama-mountain-music-lyrics

Blue Bell ice cream commercial late 1980s. YouTube, uploaded by Dallas VHS closet on June 27, 2014, https://youtu.be/54XHWdE0kq8?si=_QvVAG0w1sgcaSOQ

Reed, Jerry / Rose, Deena Kaye. Lyrics to "East Bound and Down". RCA Records, 1977. Genius.com, https://genius.com/Jerry-reed-east-bound-and-down-lyrics

Nicks, Stevie. Lyrics to "Landslide". Reprise, 1975. Genius.com, https://genius.com/Fleetwood-mac-landslide-lyrics

Hartford, John. Lyrics to "Gentle On My Mind". Capitol, 1967. Genius.com, https://genius.com/Glen-campbell-gentle-on-my-mind-lyrics

Perry, Bill / Buck, Peter / Mills, Mike / Stipe, Michael. Lyrics to "It's the End of the World as We Know It (And I Feel Fine)". I.R.S, 1987. Genius.com, https://genius.com/Rem-its-the-end-of-the-world-as-we-know-it-and-i-feel-fine-lyrics

Schönberg, Claude-Michel / Kretzmer, Herbert. Lyrics to "I Dreamed a Dream". Universal Republic, 1980. Genius.com, https://genius.com/Claude-michel-schonberg-i-dreamed-a-dream-lyrics

Brumley, Albert E. Lyrics to "I'll Fly Away". Hartford Music Company, 1932. Genius.com, https://genius.com/Gillian-welch-and-alison-krauss-ill-fly-away-lyrics

The Outback Diaries

213

Also by Randy Tharp

The Outback Diaries
Artificial Monsters

Watch for more at https://tharpster.org/.

About the Author

Randy Tharp keeps the memories of his youth and formative years tucked away in Casper, Wyoming, where the seasons are distinct and the wind never takes a day off. He now resides in Texas, the state of his birth, where he's living out the post-formative years of life. He's been married for over 30 years, is the proud father of two grown children, grandfather to one endlessly curious grandson, and currently training Tonka—the family's recently adopted Weimaraner with boundless energy.

By day, Randy works as a Business Analyst in the financial services industry, where he spends his time navigating spreadsheets, meetings, and mastering the ancient corporate art of looking busy. Outside of work, he writes when he has something to say, reads when something grabs his interest, and updates his blog at Tharpster.Org whenever a topic won't leave him alone.

Read more at https://tharpster.org/.